KU-227-465

Manual of Respiratory Care Procedures

Diane Blodgett, C.R.T.T., R.R.T.

Technical Director
Respiratory Therapy
Faxton Hospital
Children's Hospital and
Rehabilitation Center
Utica, New York

CHESTER COLLEGE

ACC. No.	DEPT.
01005780	

CLASS No.

616-2004636 BLO

LIBRARY

J. B. Lippincott Company
Philadelphia • Toronto

Copyright © 1980, by J. B. Lippincott Company

This book is fully protected by copyright, and with the exception of brief excerpts for review, no part of it may be reproduced in any form, by print, photoprint, microfilm, or any other means, without written permission from the publisher.

ISBN 0-397-50434-9

Library of Congress Catalog Card Number 79-22601

Printed in the United States

1 3 5 6 4 2

Library of Congress Cataloging in Publication Data

Blodgett, Diane.
  Manual of respiratory care procedures.

  1. Inhalation therapy—Handbooks, manuals, etc.
I. Title.
RC735.I5B56   616.2'004'636   79-22601
ISBN 0-397-50434-9

TO
Dr. Malcom Gilbert, my Respiratory Therapy Mentor,
Jeffrey, Lisa, and Nathan, my Life Mentors

Contributors

Terry Houts, B.S., R.R.T.
Formerly Director, Respiratory Therapy
Barnes Hospital
St. Louis, Missouri

Robert Fluck, B.S., R.R.T.
Instructor
Respiratory Therapy Programs
College of Health Related Professions
State University of New York
Upstate Medical Center
Syracuse, New York

Frank Smith, B.S., R.R.T.
Assistant Professor
Clinical Coordinator
Respiratory Therapy Programs
College of Health Related Professions
State University of New York
Upstate Medical Center
Syracuse, New York

Carl Wiezalis, M.S., R.R.T.
Program Director
Respiratory Therapy Programs
College of Health Related Professions
State University of New York
Upstate Medical Center
Syracuse, New York

Preface

I undertook this project to provide the respiratory care practitioner with a guide to use at the bedside. Textbooks are left in the library, procedure manuals, in the technical director's office, and a helpful formula learned in a lecture, left on a pad somewhere in a locker. It was thus obvious to me that the practitioner needed a handbook that he could carry with him.

It is suggested, then, that the practitioner and student alike carry this procedure handbook with them—use it, write in it, revise it, and delete and add to it. I am not suggesting that all the information you need for your day to day respiratory care practice is here. I do, however, provide the reader with useful guidelines and procedures.

PLEASE WRITE IN THIS BOOK

It is for you, the respiratory practitioner.

There are areas that this book does not cover—primarily pediatrics—that must be addressed separately.

This guide, should, however, provide most of the information needed in the clinical environment.

Acknowledgments

Though there will be some I will miss, the following people contributed more than many of them realize.

Thanks to Jeffrey, Lisa, and Nathan, who have missed me for the last year, but managed to keep the home fires burning. To my mother and sisters, who show pride in my accomplishments. To Marilyn Stern, Ginny VanLeuven, Ruth Groesbeck, Annette Sharkey, who typed many pages and typed them again and again. To Barbara, who drew the illustrations again and just once more. To my staff, especially Larry, who stuck around through thick and thin. To Mr. Richard Warren, my boss, who I will never be able to thank enough for the encouragement and help I seem to have needed and which he gave freely. To my contributors, Frank, Bob, Terry and Carl, who lightened the burden.

Introduction to Clinical Respiratory Care

Three of the essential components in the delivery of respiratory therapy are the patient, the procedure, and the outcome. Most of this book addresses the procedures. This introduction discusses the patient and the outcome of our procedures. But we, the practitioners, are directly involved with all three.

First, you should want to know the following.

The Patient
1. Who the patient is.
2. What his medical problem is, especially the problem that is requiring your intervention.

The Procedure
3. What did the physician have in mind when he ordered respiratory therapy? Did he make the appropriate choice? Will the procedure help achieve the objectives of our care?

The Outcome
4. What should the outcome of our care be? How can we evaluate the outcome?

What we must know about our patient are the facts that will affect our interaction with him. Some facts will be obvious when we enter the room; male or female, old or young. Other data must be obtained from the chart: the diagnosis, history and physical, lab results, etc. Finally, more information can be learned from the patient himself, through dialogue and examination. It is important to evaluate your patient before proceeding with respiratory care.

The information about the patient will help you decide therapeutic objectives. In each chapter of this book, the therapeutic objectives for each treatment modality are provided.

If the patient has a history of left lower lobe pneumonia, which is then verified by physical findings and x-ray, then the objective is *to clear the pneumonia.* How do we accomplish that? The orders should be written so that the procedure used will achieve our goal. In this case, it might be ultrasonic nebulizer for 15 min. with ½ normal saline, followed by chest physiotherapy to include clapping and postural drainage to left lower lobe 4 times a day. Once the physician has written the orders appropriate to achieving the goal, then the therapy is given following standards of care for that treatment modality. At this time, it is also appropriate to identify the criteria for termination of the therapy. How will we know when to stop? "Death or discharge" is never appropriate. The following form, completed during the initial evaluation, helps the therapist to identify the pertinent information about the respiratory care to be given (See Evaluation Form).

To provide the best care to respiratory patients, the respiratory practitioner must pay special care when performing procedures. We must have a good grasp of the procedure, the benefits, side effects, and hazards. We should explain the therapy to our patient, to obtain full cooperation. As we administer therapy, we should observe the patient for changes. We should use all our resources in order to maximize the benefits to the patient.

Once we know about the patient, and procedure has been followed, we must evaluate the care we have given. Did the patient improve, remain unchanged, or get worse? How do we evaluate our patient? Each section of the book follows a format that states an objective and provides a guide to a procedure. Our first procedure sets a standard for the evaluation of the therapy. *Objective:* To evaluate the respiratory care method used to treat primary pulmonary disease or secondary pulmonary complications.

Procedure: Based on the specific problem that the patient may have, the following means of evaluation should be used.

A. Oxygenation. The respiratory therapist can superficially evaluate oxygenation by checking vital signs and inspecting the lips, tongue, and extremities for signs of cyanosis. Because cyanosis may not be obvious in all patients, arterial blood gas sampling is the method of choice for evaluating oxygenation. Oxygen therapy dosage can not be titrated unless an arterial blood gas sample is analyzed.

B. Ventilation. Auscultation gives the respiratory therapist an

THE FAXTON HOSPITAL
and
CHILDREN'S HOSPITAL AND REHABILITATION CENTER
Department of Respiratory Therapy
Evaluation Form

Patient's Name: _____ Room # _____ Date: _____

Age: _____ Diagnosis _____

_____

Therapeutic objectives of Respiratory Care: _____

_____

_____

Respiratory Care instructions necessary to achieve objectives

(type Rx, frequency, duration, and medication): _____

_____

_____

_____

_____

Criteria for termination of Respiratory Care: _____

_____

_____

_____

Respiratory Care Record (see attached forms).

Initiate Therapy:

Signature: _____

Date: _____

easy method of evaluating whether or not the patient is moving air throughout the lung fields. For those patients with primary lung disease, a simple spirometry (FVC, FEV$_1$) before and after therapy can indicate whether or not there is improvement. For those patients with respiratory insufficiency or failure, arterial blood gas values are the *most* conclusive means of evaluating ventilation before and after therapy (Pa$_{CO_2}$ = ventilation).

C. Humidity and Aerosol Therapy. Sputum viscosity can be evaluated by comparing pretherapy sputum viscosity with post-therapy viscosity. Color change (*i.e.*, from yellow to clear) can also indicate improvement. The ability of the patient to clear his airway and mobilize secretions is another means of evaluating the effectiveness of aerosol therapy. Evaluation by auscultation is also indicated on the overall examination determining the result of therapy.

The therapist must also know how to identify an adverse reaction. We now come to our second procedure: how to identify an adverse reaction to therapy.

Objective: To identify an adverse reaction. Once the adverse reaction has been identified, to take the appropriate action.

Procedure: Guidelines for identification of an adverse reaction during respiratory treatment.

1. The therapist should monitor changes in vital signs for
   a. Change in pulse
   b. Change in blood pressure
   c. Change in respiration rate
   d. Change in level of consciousness
2. The therapist should monitor changes in physical signs for
   a. Diaphoresis
   b. Cyanosis
   c. Increase work of breathing
   d. Nausea, vomiting
   e. Vertigo
   f. Decrease or change in breath sounds

Once adverse reaction has been identified, the therapist should look for the possible cause: bronchospasm, pneumothorax, cardiac arrest, bronchodilator overdose, improper teaching of Rx. When that is accomplished, take the appropriate action.

If there are adverse changes in vital signs, the therapist should
   a. Stop Rx.
   b. Report changes in vital signs to head nurse.

   c. Stay with the patient until vital signs normalize.

   d. Chart adverse reaction and vital signs in patient's respiratory care record.

If there are adverse changes in physical signs, the therapist should

   a. Stop Rx—stay with patient until stable.

   b. Inform head nurse.

   c. Administer O_2 for cyanosis or increased work of breathing.

   d. Maintain clear airway and initiate CPR, if necessary.

   e. Chart adverse change in patient's respiratory care record.

If, in the therapist's opinion, the adverse reaction is serious, or life threatening, he should seek a physician's assistance immediately.

Finally, once we know about the patient, have given the therapy and evaluated the outcome, documentation is essential. We must communicate the information we have to other members of the health care team. The respiratory care record should include the date, the time therapy was administered, the results of therapy, and the signature of the practitioner administering the care. The results of therapy should include vital signs: pre-, during and post-therapy, breath sounds, notation about sputum production and/or cough and an overall evaluation of the therapy (oxygenation, ventilation and humidity and aerosol therapy).

If the patient refuses or is unavailable for therapy (*e.g.,* in x-ray), it should be noted.

If the patient has an adverse reaction, it should be documented, along with the critical management. Results of tests performed by the technician or therapist should also be documented in the chart.

If we do all of these things—examine the patient, perform therapy according to accepted standards of respiratory care, evaluate the results of our care, and document what we do and the patient outcome—we are meeting the objectives of our profession, which are to provide the patient with optimum care.

Contents

Appendices

CHAPTER ONE

Gas Administration Devices
Diane Blodgett, R.R.T.

General Considerations for Gas Administration

This section deals with the delivery of therapeutic gases. The gases that are generally given by the Respiratory Therapist are *Oxygen* and combinations of *Oxygen* and *Carbon Dioxide* or *Oxygen* and *Helium*.

The therapeutic objectives for *oxygen* administration are decrease in myocardial work, decrease in respiratory work and relief or prevention of hypoxia. Hypoxia is the primary indication for the administration of oxygen. The etiology of hypoxia may involve an insufficient amount of oxygen crossing the alveolar capillary membrane (hypoxic hypoxia), an inability of blood to accept and transport sufficient oxygen (hemic hypoxia), a blood flow insufficient to provide oxygen to the tissues (stagnant hypoxia), an inability to utilize the oxygen at the tissue level (histotoxic hypoxia), and finally, an inability to supply sufficient oxygen to meet the demand (demand hypoxia). The type of disease and the degree of hypoxia will determine the appropriate concentration and device that should be used.

There are essentially no contraindications to the use of O_2; however, there are some hazards that accompany its use, especially when that use is excessive. These hazards include loss of hypoxic drive in the patient who chronically retains carbon dioxide, and oxygen toxicity in patients who receive high levels of oxygen over a prolonged period of time—it can occur in less than 24 hours. The CO_2 retainer will appear lethargic, confused, somnolent, and will have shallow respirations. ABGs will reveal respiratory acidosis with or without hypoxemia. The patient with oxygen toxicity might complain of substernal pain, headache,

1

Table 1-1. Gas Administration

Gases	Indications	Disease Entities	Gas Concentrations	Devices to Administer Gas
Oxygen	1. Stagnant hypoxia	Shock Heart failure	35-100%	Catheter Cannula Simple mask Partial rebreathing mask
	2. Histoxic	Cyanide poisoning	35-100%, depending on severity	Catheter Cannula All masks
	3. Hemic hypoxia	Anemia Hemorrhage CO poisoning Methemoglobinemia	100%	Non-rebreathing mask
	4. Hypoxic hypoxia	High Altitude Suffocation Drowning Pulmonary Edema COPD	24-100%	Catheter Cannula All masks

	5. Demand hypoxia	Fever Exercise	24-40%	Catheter Cannula Simple mask
Carbon dioxide/oxygen	1. Increase cerebral blood flow	CVA	95% Oxygen 5% Carbon Dioxide	Non-rebreathing mask
	2. Hyperinflation of lungs	Atelectasis		
	3. Hiccups			
Helium/oxygen	1. Large airway obstruction	Tumor obstructing bronchus	70% Helium/30% Oxygen 80% Helium/20% Oxygen	Non-rebreathing mask

[3]

cough, and even dyspnea. Absorption atelectasis may appear. ABGs will reveal a high Pa_{O_2}. The criteria for termination of O_2 therapy are a stable cardio-vascular system, acceptable blood gases on room air and the elimination of the underlying disease causing hypoxia.

The therapeutic objectives for the administration of a mixture of *oxygen* and *carbon dioxide* are the increase of cerebral blood flow, induction of hyperinflation and treatment of hiccups. Mixtures of CO_2 (5%)/O_2 (95%) are usually administered intermittently (*i.e.*, QID) by non-rebreathing mask. The primary contraindication to O_2–CO_2 therapy is a patient's chronic CO_2 retention. The hazards include headache, depression, acute changes in vital signs (tachycardia, hypertension), and possibly seizures and cardiac arrest. The criteria for the termination of therapy are the improvement in cerebral blood flow, the ability of the patient to hyperinflate his lungs voluntarily and the cessation of hiccups.

The therapeutic objective for the administration of *oxygen* and *helium* is the relief of large airway obstruction. Mixtures of He (70%)/O_2 (30%) and He (80%)/O_2 (20%) are usually administered continuously by non-rebreathing mask. There are no contraindications to the administration of O_2/He mixtures. If high concentrations of oxygen are necessary, however, then the small concentration of He that might be added will be of little benefit. Concentrations of 70-80% helium are the most beneficial. Because helium is a safe, inert gas, there is only a minor problem with its administration and that is the change in voice tone. The criterion for termination of therapy is the decrease in airway obstruction.

OXYGEN CATHETER

Description

Oxygen catheter is a smooth, flexible tube, approximately 16 inches in length. The catheter has multiple, well spaced openings on the patient end.

Objective

To administer low to moderate concentrations of oxygen nasally.

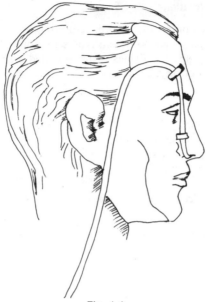

Fig. 1-1.

Procedure

1. Approach the patient and explain the procedure.

2. To determine the insertion depth of the catheter, measure the distance from the patient's external nares to the end of the ear lobe.

3. With the humidifier, tubing and catheter connected, set the oxygen flow at a low rate.

4. Lubricate the catheter with a water-soluble lubricant. Check gas flow.

5. Determine the natural droop of the catheter.

6. With the oxygen still at low flow, insert the catheter along the floor of the nasal passage to the measured depth. Check placement by depressing tongue; if catheter is seen opposite uvula, pull back slightly (¼ in.).

7. Use adhesive strips to tape the catheter firmly to the side of the nose.

8. Adjust oxygen to desired flow.

9. Clip tubing to the bed sheet after allowing enough slack for the patient to move his head.

Special Considerations

- Place O_2 sign on entrance to patient's room.
- *Encourage* physician to obtain ABGs to monitor Pa_{O_2}.
- No smoking, sparks, flames or ungrounded electrical equipment in area of oxygen use.

Hazards

- Nasal irritation.
- Drying of the nasal mucosa.
- Possible gastric distention.
- Epistaxis.

Flows and Inspired O_2 Concentrations

Liter Flows
  1-6 LPM yield O_2 concentrations of 22-50%. This is dependent upon patient's ventilatory pattern.

Maintenance

- Every eight hours at most, remove catheter and insert new one in alternate nostril, if possible.
- Discard catheter and tubing after use.

SMALL-BORE TUBING WITH CANNULA

Description

Over-the-ear nasal oxygen cannula is a bifurcated, flexible tube that directs the oxygen flow into the nose by means of two plastic tips which fit into the nostrils.

Objective

To administer low to moderate oxygen concentrations nasally.

Procedure

1. Approach the patient and explain the procedure.
2. With the humidifier, tubing and cannula connected, set the oxygen flow at a low rate.
3. Insert tips of cannula in nostrils.
4. Slip the two smaller plastic tubes over the ears and under

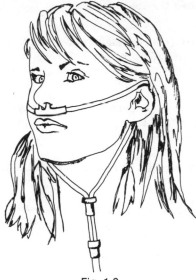

Fig. 1-2.

the chin. Adjust the plastic slide until the cannula fits snugly and comfortably.

    5. Clip tubing to clothes after allowing enough slack for patient to turn head.

    6. Adjust oxygen flow to rate specified in doctor's orders.

Special Considerations

- Place O_2 sign on entrance to patient's room.
- *Encourage* physician to obtain ABGs to monitor Pa_{O_2}.
- Nasal prongs may be cut shorter if uncomfortable for patient.
- This method of administration is effective only if the nasal passages are unobstructed.
- No smoking, sparks, flames or ungrounded electrical equipment in area of oxygen use.

Hazards

- Nasal irritation.
- Drying of the nasal mucosa.
- Sinus pain.
- Epistaxis.

Flows and Inspired O₂ Concentrations

Liter Flows
1-6 LPM yield O_2 concentrations of 22-50%. This is dependent upon patient's ventilatory pattern.

Maintenance

- Check the position of cannula tips frequently.
- Discard cannula and tubing after use.

SMALL-BORE TUBING AND SIMPLE MASK

Description

Simple mask is a flexible cone-shaped device. It has metal strip to mold the mask to the nose, an adjustable head strap and multiple exhalation ports.

Objective

To deliver medium concentrations of oxygen by mask.

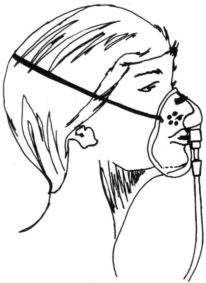

Fig. 1-3.

Procedure

1. Approach the patient and explain the procedure.
2. With the humidifier, tubing and mask connected, set the oxygen at a low flow rate.
3. Carefully adjust headband so the fit is snug, but not too tight.
4. Adjust the metal strip on the nose portion and mold mask to face.
5. Adjust O_2 flow to desired level.

Special Considerations

- Place O_2 sign on entrance to patient's room.
- *Encourage* physician to obtain ABGs to monitor Pa_{O_2}.
- Flow must be 3-4 LPM to eliminate CO_2.
- No smoking, sparks, flames or ungrounded electrical equipment in area of oxygen use.

Hazards

- Aspiration with vomiting patient.
- CO_2 accumulation at low flow rate.
- Subcutaneous emphysema into ocular tissue at high flow rate.
- Pressure necrosis with tight fitting masks.

Flows and Inspired O_2 Concentrations

Liter Flows
    3-10 LPM yield O_2 concentrations of 25-55%.

Maintenance

- Adjust mask PRN.
- Discard mask and tubing after use.

PARTIAL REBREATHING MASK WITH SMALL-BORE TUBING

Description

A partial rebreathing mask is a flexible cone-shaped device with a reservoir bag attached. It has a metal strip to mold the mask to the nose, and an adjustable head strap, but differs from

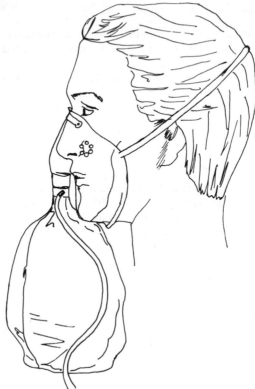

Fig. 1-4.

the non-rebreathing mask by not having one-way flap valves between bag and mask and on the exhalation ports.

Objective

To administer medium to medium-high concentrations of oxygen by mask with reservoir bag.

Procedure

1. Approach the patient and explain the procedure.
2. With the humidifier, tubing and mask connected, set the oxygen flow at a low rate.
3. Fill the reservoir bag with oxygen by occluding opening between bag and mask.

4. Slip strap around head.

5. Carefully adjust headband so the fit is snug, but not too tight.

6. Adjust the metal strip on the nose portion and mold mask to face.

7. Adjust oxygen flow so the bag will fill on exhalation and then *almost* collapse on inspiration.

8. Adjust flow to higher rate, if necessary.

Special Considerations

- Place O_2 sign on entrance to patient's room.
- *Encourage* physician to obtain ABGs to monitor Pa_{O_2}.
- No smoking, sparks, flames or ungrounded electrical equipment in area of oxygen use.

Hazards

- Aspiration with vomiting patient.
- Pressure necrosis with tight fitting mask.
- Subcutaneous emphysema into ocular tissue at very high flows.
- CO_2 accumulation at low flows.

Flows and Inspired O_2 Concentrations

Liter Flows

O_2 concentration of 35-60% can be achieved by adjusting flows to patient needs. The better the mask fit the higher the concentration.

Maintenance

- If bag accumulates water, empty water out.
- Discard mask and tubing after use.

NON-REBREATHING MASK

Description

A non-rebreathing mask is a flexible cone-shaped device with a reservoir bag attached. It has a metal strip to mold the mask to the nose, an adjustable head strap, a flap valve between bag and mask, and flap valves on the exhalation ports.

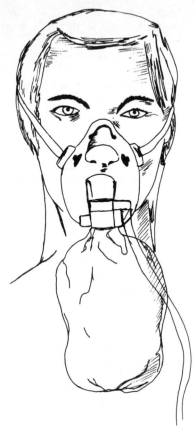

Fig. 1-5.

Objective

To administer high concentrations of oxygen by mask with reservoir bag.

Procedure

1. Approach the patient and explain the procedure.
2. With the humidifier, tubing and mask connected, set the oxygen flow at a low rate.
3. Fill the reservoir bag with oxygen by occluding the one way valve between bag and mask.
4. Slip strap around head.

5. Carefully adjust headband so the fit is snug, but not too tight.

6. Adjust the metal strip on the nose portion and mold mask to face.

7. Adjust oxygen flow so that the bag will fill on expiration and then *almost* collapse on inspiration.

8. Adjust flow to higher rate, if necessary.

Special Considerations

- Place O_2 sign on entrance to patient's room.
- *Encourage* physician to obtain ABGs to monitor Pa_{O_2}.
- Make sure flap valves are not sticking.
- No smoking, sparks, flames or ungrounded electrical equipment in area of oxygen use.

Hazards

- Aspiration with vomiting patient.
- Subcutaneous emphysema into ocular tissue at very high flows.
- Pressure necrosis with tight fitting masks.
- Suffocation due to insufficient flow.
- CO_2 accumulation at low flows.

Flows and Inspired O_2 Concentrations

The oxygen concentrations will be high; the better the mask fit, the higher the concentration.

Concentrations of 95% + 5% can be achieved.

Flows must be sufficient to meet the patient's inspiratory demands.

Maintenance

- If bag accumulates water, empty water out.
- Discard mask and tubing after use.

SMALL-BORE TUBING WITH VENTURIMASK

Description

Venturimask is a cone-shaped device with entrainment ports of various sizes at the base of the mask. It has a metal strip to mold the mask to the nose, an adjustable head strap and multiple exhalation ports.

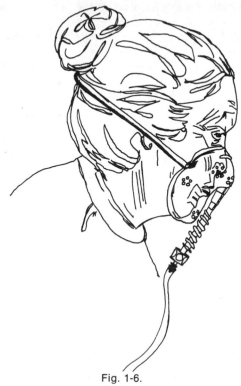

Fig. 1-6.

Objective

To give a prescribed precise low-medium concentration of oxygen by mask.

Procedure

1. Approach the patient and explain the procedure.
2. Attach tubing directly to flowmeter for low-concentration masks. Use humidifier for higher-concentration masks.
3. Adjust the flow of oxygen to that stated on the mask.
4. Slip strap around head.
5. Adjust the metal strip on the nose portion and mold mask to face.
6. Carefully adjust headband so the fit is snug, but not too tight.

Special Considerations

- Place O_2 sign on entrance to patient's room.
- *Encourage* physician to obtain ABGs to monitor Pa_{O_2}.
- Be careful that venturi openings are always clear.
- No smoking, sparks, flames or ungrounded electrical equipment in area of oxygen use.

Hazards

- Aspiration with vomiting patient.
- Pressure necrosis with tight-fitting mask.
- Subcutaneous emphysema into ocular tissue at very high flows.

Flows and Inspired O_2 Concentrations (See Table 1-2)

Table 1-2.
Flows and Inspired O_2 Concentrations of Common Venturi-Masks.

Mask%	Liter Flow	Air/O_2	Total Flow
24	4	20:1	84 LPM
28	4	10:1	44 LPM
31	6	7:1	49 LPM
35	8	5:1	48 LPM
40	8	3:1	32 LPM

Maintenance

- Maintain flow as indicated on mask.
- Discard mask and tubing after use.

AEROSOL MASK

Description

An aerosol mask is a flexible cone-shaped device. It has a metal strip to mold the mask to the nose, an adjustable head strap, two large openings for exhalation and a large bore tubing connection.

Objective

To administer, by mask, oxygen or air-oxygen mixtures saturated with water vapor at body temperature.

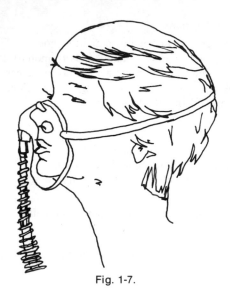

Fig. 1-7.

Procedure

1. Approach patient and explain the procedure.

2. With the nebulizer, tubing and mask connected, set the gas flow at 10 LPM.

3. Slip strap around head.

4. Carefully adjust headband so the fit is snug, but not too tight.

5. Adjust the metal strip on the hose portion and mold mask to face.

6. Readjust flow to meet patient's needs. Mist should always be visible.

Special Considerations

- Make sure flow is adequate (mist visible).
- If oxygen is carrier gas, *encourage* physician to obtain ABGs to monitor Pa_{O_2}.
- If oxygen is carrier gas, place O_2 sign on entrance to patient's room.
- Since output is high with nebulizer, make sure tubing is not blocked by water.
- No smoking, sparks, flames or ungrounded electrical equipment in area of oxygen use.

Hazards

- Water accumulation in tubing.
- Aspiration with vomiting patient.
- Pressure necrosis with tight fitting mask.

Flows and Inspired O₂ Concentrations

Concentrations are stable when a venturi nebulizer is used at high flow rates. Concentrations delivered can be from 21–100%, depending on nebulizer settings.

Maintenance

- Keep jar filled with sterile distilled water.
- Drain water when necessary.
- Wipe accumulated moisture from inside of mask when necessary.
- Discard tubing and mask after use.

FACE TENT

Description

The face tent is a shield-like device that fits under the chin and sweeps around the face. It has an adjustable head strap and large bore tubing connection.

Objective

To administer oxygen or air-oxygen mixtures saturated with water vapor at body temperature.

Procedure

1. Approach the patient and explain the procedure.

2. With the nebulizer, tubing and face tent connected, set the gas flow at 10 LPM (nebulizer setting will determine F_{IO_2}).

3. Slip strap around head and place tent under chin.

4. Carefully adjust headband so the fit is snug, but not too tight.

5. Readjust flow to meet patient's needs. Mist should always be visible.

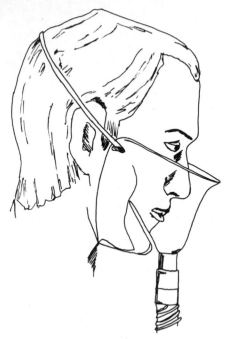

Fig. 1-8.

Special Considerations

- Make sure flow is adequate (mist visible).
- If oxygen is carrier gas, *encourage* physician to obtain ABGs to monitor Pa_{O_2}.
- If oxygen is carrier gas, place O_2 sign on entrance to patient's room.
- Since output is high with nebulizer, make sure tubing is not blocked by water accumulation.
- No smoking, sparks, flames or ungrounded electrical equipment in area of oxygen use.

Hazards

- Water accumulation in tubing.

Flows and Inspired O₂ Concentrations

Concentrations are stable when a venturi nebulizer is used at high flow rates. Concentrations delivered can be from 21–80%, depending on nebulizer setting.

Maintenance

- Keep jar filled with sterile distilled water.
- Drain water when necessary.
- Discard tubing and T-tube after use.

TRACH MASK

Description

Trach mask is a flexible collar-shaped device with an adjustable neck strap, large bore tubing connection and large exhalation port.

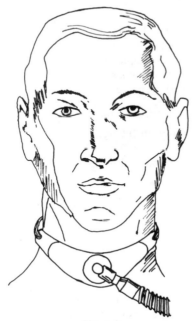

Fig. 1-9.

Objective

To deliver oxygen or air-oxygen mixtures saturated with water vapor at body temperature to the patient with a tracheostomy or laryngectomy.

Procedure

1. Approach the patient and explain the procedure.
2. With the nebulizer, tubing and trach mask attached, set the gas flow at 10 LPM (nebulizer setting will determine $F_{I_{O_2}}$).
3. Slip strap around patient's neck.
4. Adjust strap so mask lies loosely in front to meet patient's needs.
5. Readjust flow to meet patient's needs.

Special Considerations

- Make sure flow is adequate (mist visible).
- If oxygen is carrier gas, *encourage* physician to obtain ABGs to monitor Pa_{O_2}.
- If oxygen is carrier gas, place O_2 sign on entrance to patient's room.
- Heating the mist is advisable.
- Since output is high with nebulizer, make sure tubing is not blocked by water accumulation.
- No smoking, sparks, flames or ungrounded electrical equipment in area of oxygen use.

Hazards

- Water accumulation in tubing.
- Infection
- Pulmonary and/or tracheal burns when aerosol is heated.
- Local irritation.

Flows and Inspired O_2 Concentrations

Concentrations are fairly stable when a venturi nebulizer is used at high flow rates. Concentrations delivered can be from 21–100% depending on nebulizer setting.

Maintenance

- Keep jar filled with sterile distilled water.
- Drain water when necessary.
- Discard tubing and trach mask after use.

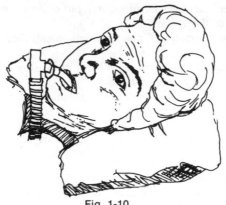

Fig. 1-10.

AEROSOL T-TUBE

Description

Plastic T-adaptor that fits directly to tracheostomy or endotracheal tubes that have 15mm connections. Large bore tubing is used to transmit the aerosol from its generator to the T-tube.

Objective

To administer oxygen or air-oxygen mixtures saturated with water-vapor at body temperature.

Procedure

1. Approach the patient and explain the procedure.
2. With the nebulizer, tubing and T-tube connected, set the gas flow at 10 LPM (nebulizer setting will determine F_{IO_2}).
3. Attach the T-tube to the endotracheal tube or tracheostomy tube.
4. Readjust flow to meet patient's needs. Mist should always be visible.

Special Considerations

• Add reservoir tube on exhalation side of T-tube to maintain stable oxygen concentration.
• Make sure flow is adequate (mist visible).
• Heating the mist is advisable.

- If oxygen is carrier gas, *encourage* physician to obtain ABGs to monitor Pa_{O_2}.
- If oxygen is carrier gas, place O_2 sign on entrance to patient's room.
- Since output is high with nebulizer, make sure tubing is not blocked by water accumulation.
- No smoking, sparks, flames or ungrounded electrical equipment in area of oxygen use.

Hazards

- Water accumulation in tubing.
- Overhydration.
- Pulmonary and/or tracheal burns when aerosol is heated.
- Blockage of T-tube with secretions.
- Infection.

Flows and Inspired O_2 Concentrations

Concentrations are stable when a venturi nebulizer is used at high flow rates. Concentrations delivered can be from 21–100% depending on nebulizer setting.

Maintenance

- Keep jar filled with sterile distilled water.
- Drain water when necessary.
- Discard tubing and T-tube after use.

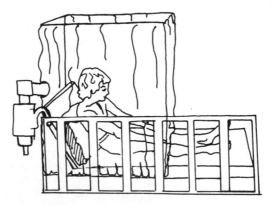

Fig. 1-11.

AEROSOL TENT (CROUPETTE)

Description

The aerosol tent is an enclosure device that consists of a plastic canopy, a cooling and/or circulating unit and a nebulizer.

Objective

To provide a high-humidity environment, with or without oxygen enrichment, cooled to 6-15° below ambient. Its primary application is for infants or youths who will not accept other gas administration devices.

Procedure

1. Approach the patient and explain the procedure.
2. Position cooling nebulizer unit on crib or bed.
3. Attach canopy to unit and position over bed.
4. Fill ice chamber or start refrigeration unit.
5. Fill nebulizer reservoir with sterile distilled water.
6. Set flow through nebulizer to at least 10 LPM (source gas and nebulizer dilution will determine F_{IO_2}).
7. Place patient in tent.
8. Tuck in canopy sides under mattress. Fold sheet over front portion of the tent edge.
9. Adjust flow when patient is settled.

Special Considerations

- Make sure gas flow is sufficient.
- Keep canopy tucked in and closed to maintain stable environment.
- If oxygen is used as carrier gas, monitor F_{IO_2}, either continuously or q4h.
- If oxygen is carrier gas, place O_2 sign on entrance to patient's room.
- No smoking, sparks, flames or ungrounded electrical equipment in area of oxygen use.
- No friction toys in tent.

Hazards

- CO_2 accumulation at low flow.
- Unstable oxygen concentrations when enclosure is opened.

- Fire with supplementary oxygen.
- With high-humidity atmosphere (using high-output nebulizer), fluid overload and loss of patient visibility are possible hazards.

Flows and Inspired O₂ Concentrations

Concentrations of 21–60% are obtainable, depending on flow rate and tightness of enclosure.

Maintenance

- Keep nebulizer jar filled with sterile distilled water.
- Ice chamber must be kept filled with a combination of ice and water.
- Bedding and patient clothes may need frequent changing as a result of dampness.

Primary Gas Source Devices

This section deals with the equipment that supplies the therapeutic gases. Tanks, compressors, piping systems, concentrators, blenders and the equipment that controls the pressure and flow of gas are all covered in the following procedures.

In the previous section, the therapeutic uses of various gases, gas mixtures, and the devices necessary to administer the gases were presented. Now we need to know how to use and control the sources of gas that we use. In some instances, it is a less complex piece of equipment, such as a compressor or concentrator that supplies the gas. The more complicated system may include obtaining two gas sources and using a blender to deliver a precise mixture of air and oxygen.

Whatever the source gas, the procedures for its use and the necessary safety standards that must be followed are reviewed in this section.

TANKS-CYLINDERS

Description

Cylinders and tanks for medical gas usage are supplied in sizes from AA to H or K. These gas sources are used to supply medical gases in a portable container to the patient. The tanks are gen-

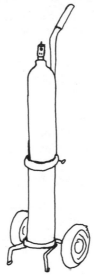

Fig. 1-12.

erally color coded, have markings that identify their contents, and have standardized valve outlet fittings (see Tables 1-3 and 1-4).

Color Coding for Cylinders

OXYGEN (O_2)—Green
CARBON DIOXIDE (CO_2)—Gray
CARBON DIOXIDE/OXYGEN (CO_2/O_2)—Gray/Green
NITROUS OXIDE (N_2O)—Blue
HELIUM (He)—Brown
HELIUM/OXYGEN (He/O_2)—Brown/Green
CYCLOPRAPANE (C_3H_6)—Orange
ETHYLENE (C_2H_4)—Red
NITROGEN (N_2)—Black
NITROGEN/OXYGEN (N_2/O_2)—Black/Green

Gas Categories

OXYGEN—Oxidant
CARBON DIOXIDE—Inert
CYCLOPROPANE—Flammable
ETHYLENE-ETHYLENE OXIDE—Flammable
HELIUM—Inert
NITROGEN—Inert
NITROUS OXIDE—Oxident

Objective

To provide medical gases in a portable unit.

Procedure

The following procedures are used in conjunction with medical gas cylinders.

General Storage Procedures

1. Storage must follow all National Fire Prevention Association regulations. Local regulations and codes may further restrict storage of gases.
2. Separate flammable gases from all other gases (store in separate areas).
3. Store full and empty cylinders separately.
4. Store oxygen and nitrous oxide in a well-vented (to the outside), cool, dry and fire-resistant area.
5. Provision must be made so that tanks cannot be knocked over.
   a. Chained to wall for larger cylinders.
   b. Racks for smaller cylinders.
6. Do not store cylinders in the operating room.
7. Store cylinders so they are protected from extreme weather conditions.
8. Caps should be kept in place during storage.

Transportation—in-hospital guidelines

1. Tanks should be transported on carts provided for that use.
2. Transport tanks in the upright position.
3. Secure the tank with chain or strap onto the cart.
4. Push the cart so you can have maximum handling abilities (do not pull).

Usage—in-hospital guidelines

1. Cylinders must always be cracked to remove lint or soil from the cylinder outlet. Crack tank away from you.
2. Turn tanks on slowly to dissipate heat. Open valve fully and back ¼ turn.
3. Never let oil, grease or fuel of any type come in contact with cylinder valves or regulators.
4. Post "No Smoking" signs on tanks and directly outside the room where oxygen is in use. No open flames, sparks or smoking should occur in this area.
5. When oxygen is in use with a controlled environment de-

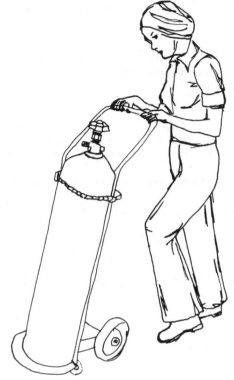

Fig. 1-13. Four-wheel cart.

vice, do not use electrical or battery operated equipment or toys (*i.e.*, call bells, TV control, friction toys).

   6. Test for leaks with solution of soapy water.

Special Considerations

- Read label to identify gas.
- Do not use if label cannot be read or has been removed.
- Do not depend on color coding for identification.

$$\text{E cylinder duration of flow} = \frac{0.28 \times \text{gauge pressure}}{\text{liters per minute gas flow}}$$

$$\text{H or K cylinder duration of flow} = \frac{3.14 \times \text{gauge pressure}}{\text{liters per minute gas flow}}$$

Hazards

- Fire
- Explosion
- Personnel injuries due to incorrect handling of cylinders.
- Administration of inappropriate gas if tank is not clearly identified by labeling.

Maintenance

- Any tanks that appear damaged, isolate and return to supplier.
- Keep tanks in storage areas approved and set aside for that use only.
- Follow all regulations regarding the safe use and handling of gases.
- Never attempt to repair cylinder valves or safety relief devices.
- Replace cylinders when contents read below 500 psig.

Table 1-3. Pin Index Safety System Combinations

Gas	Pin Configurations
OXYGEN	2-5
CARBON DIOXIDE/OXYGEN (less than 7%)	2-6
CARBON DIOXIDE/OXYGEN (more than 7%)	1-6
NITROUS OXIDE	3-5
HELIUM/OXYGEN (less than 80%)	2-4
HELIUM/OXYGEN (more than 80%)	4-6
CYCLOPROPANE	3-6
ETHYLENE	1-3
AIR MEDICAL	1-5

Table 1-4. Diameter Index Safety System Numbers

Gas	Connections
OXYGEN	1240
CARBON DIOXIDE	1080
CARBON DIOXIDE/OXYGEN (less than 7%)	1080
CARBON DIOXIDE/OXYGEN (more than 7%)	1200
NITROUS OXIDE	1040
HELIUM	1060

Table 1-4. Diameter Index Safety System Numbers *(Continued)*

Gas	Connections
HELIUM/OXYGEN (less than 20%)	1060
HELIUM/OXYGEN (more than 20%)	1180
CYCLOPROPANE	1100
ETHYLENE	1140
AIR MEDICAL	1160
SUCTION	1220

REDUCING VALVES—FLOWMETERS REGULATORS

Description

A full cylinder of a medical gas may have a pressure of more than 2000 psig. Before the gas from the cylinder can be used safely, a pressure reducing regulator must be attached to the cylinder. The reducing valve reduces the high pressure from a cylinder in one, two or three stages. The flowmeter which can be attached to the reducing valve is calibrated to indicate liter flow. Flowmeter can be compensated, uncompensated, or a Bourdon Gauge. A regulator is a reducing valve and flowmeter in combination.

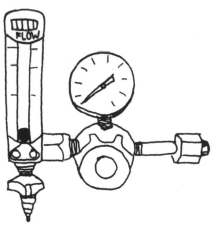

Fig. 1-14.

Objective

To reduce the high pressures in a cylinder to working pressures, and to control the rate of flow of a gas to the patient.

Procedure

The following procedures are used in conjunction with reducing valves regulator flowmeters.

Attachment of Regulator

1. Identify the cylinder by reading the label.
2. Obtain the appropriate regulator for the gas.
3. Crack cylinder to remove dust or lint from valve opening (small cylinders—remove cover seal from pin inuex configuration).
4. Attach regulator to cylinder connection and hand tighten the nut firmly. Tighten slightly with wrench if necessary. (Small cylinders: place yoke of regulator over cylinder valve. Set pins of regulator into pin holes on cylinder. Tighten wing bolt.)

Turning on Regulator

1. Open cylinder valve slowly.
2. Read contents of tank. Replace if below 500 psig.
3. Connect oxygen administrating device to flowmeter outlet.
4. Turn on flowmeter to prescribed flow rate.

Turning Off Regulator

1. Close cylinder valve slowly.
2. When flow reads zero, turn adjustment on flowmeter to the off position.

Special Considerations

- Do not use oil or grease for lubrication of regulators or flowmeters.
- Do not interchange regulators from one gas to another.
- Do not use adaptors.
- Gauges on regulators are Bourdon Gauges, indicating pressure. Thorpe tubes on regulators are either compensated or uncompensated flowmeters and indicate flows.
- Use regulators with compensated Thorpe tubes for all gas

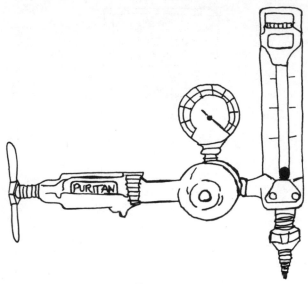

Fig. 1-15.

delivering situations except patient transport where a regulator with a Bourdon Gauge should be used. Bourdon gauges can be read in any position.
- Read flowmeter (pressure compensated) on middle of indicator ball.
- Flowmeters are usually calibrated 0-7 LPM or 0-15 LPM.
- Flowmeters can be used directly with piped systems.
- Flowmeters may incorporate high pressure outlet.

Hazards

- Fire
- Explosion
- Inaccurate flow rates with uncompensated flowmeter or Bourdon Gauge when there is back pressure.

Maintenance

- Do not use equipment that shows signs of damage or wear.
- Equipment should only be repaired by trained personnel.
- Store equipment in dust-free area.

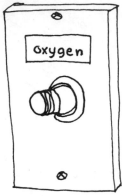

Fig. 1-16.

PIPED-GAS SOURCES-WALL OUTLETS

Description

The bulk system supplies a medical gas to the patient at the bedside. The gases that are generally provided at the bedside are oxygen, air, and vacuum. Nitrogen and nitrous oxide may be piped to the operating room also. The wall outlets should provide keyed connections so that incorrect gas administration can not be inadvertantly given. Flowmeters are used to regulate gas flow from the wall to the patient. High pressure lines provide gas source to mechanical devices such as IPPB and CMV apparatus.

Objective

To provide a compact, efficient method of administering therapeutic gases at the bedside.

Procedure

Connection of Equipment To Diameter Index Safety System (DISS) Outlets
1. Turn equipment (flowmeter/vacuum) to the off position.
2. Fasten equipment to wall outlet by twisting clockwise the female DISS adapter on to the wall male DISS adapter.
3. Turn on equipment. Adjust flowmeter or vacuum setting to appropriate position.

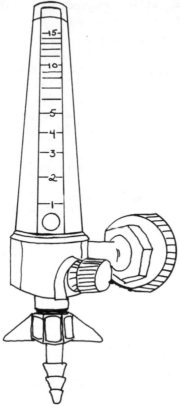

Fig. 1-17.

Disconnection of Equipment To DISS Outlets

1. Turn equipment to the off position.

2. When the indicator has dropped back to zero, unfasten the female DISS adaptor from the wall male adapter by turning counterclockwise.

3. If possible, replace dust cap on wall outlet.

Connection of Equipment to Quick-Connect Outlets

1. Close the flow adjusting valve of the flowmeter or vacuum regulator.

2. Insert the wall inlet of the flowmeter regulator into the opening of the outlet and make a firm connection.

3. Slowly open the flow adjusting valve of the flowmeter (ad-

just vacuum regulator). As the oxygen flows into the flowmeter, the float will rise. Read flow at center of ball.

Disconnection of Equipment From Quick-Connect Outlets

1. Turn equipment to the off position.
2. Release equipment from wall valve socket. Some releases are initiated by a button on wall, others by pulling retainer housing back or by pressing a release button on the housing.
3. If possible, replace dust cap on wall outlet.

Special Considerations

- Some flowmeters have a high-pressure outlet incorporated in them.
- Quick connect adapters are available in Diamond, Schrader, NCG, Puritan, OES, and Hansen Configurations. Each differs from the other slightly.
- Post "No Smoking" signs.
- Compressed air outlets may require water trap to collect condensation.

Hazards

- Contaminated piped gases.
- Low or high pressures in piping system.

Maintenance

- Report leaks in wall outlets to appropriate personnel.
- Check wall outlets periodically to make sure line pressures are being maintained at each outlet.

COMPRESSORS

Description

Devices used to provide a source of air. They are of three types: piston, diaphragm, and rotary. The compressors may provide an external or internal source of air for respiratory therapy equipment.

Objective

To provide a source of medical air to power respiratory therapy equipment.

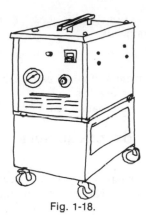

Fig. 1-18.

Procedure

Most of these devices have an on and off switch with a control knob to adjust pressure or flow.

1. Connect compressor power line to electrical outlet.
2. Connect gas-administering equipment to outlet of compressor.
3. Turn on compressor.
4. Adjust flow or pressure to meet the needs of the equipment and patient.

Special Considerations

• Choose the appropriate compressor to meet the needs of the equipment to be powered.
• Bennett, MC-1, MC-2, Ohio High Performance, Timeter PCS-1 are capable of powering a respirator and large volume output nebulizers (*i.e.*, Maxi-Cool) and can be used with blenders (*i.e.*, air-O_2 mixing devices).
• Airshields Dia-Pump, Timeter PCS-4, and DeVilbiss nebulizer compressor are capable of powering small volume output nebulizers and croupettes.
• Most compressors have oxygen DISS outlets for connection to gas administration devices.

Hazards

• Overheating
• Provision of air to patients requiring oxygen.

• Insufficient pressure or flow for needs of respiratory therapy device or patients needs.

Maintenance

• Refer to service manual if compressor cannot reach desired pressure, is noisy or overheats.
• Empty water or condensation trap PRN.

OXYGEN BLENDER

Description

Device for controlling precise oxygen concentrations to within ±3% of indicated setting. This device is operated with the use of a 50 psi air and 50 psi oxygen inlet gas pressure source. The blender is a high flow source of gas. (Some models have low-flow modules or connections.)

Objective

To deliver a precise concentration of an air-oxygen mixture through respiratory therapy equipment.

Procedure

1. Mount blender to ventilator, wall or other stable structure.
2. Connect inlet pressure hoses to blender according to the DISS connections for air and oxygen.

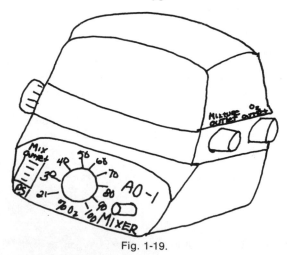

Fig. 1-19.

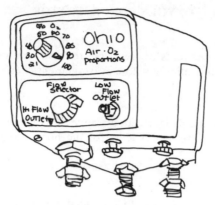

Fig. 1-20.

3. Connect each inlet hose to its separate 50 psi gas source (wall outlet or tank for oxygen and wall outlet, tank or compressor for compressed air).

4. Connect equipment to outlet fitting.

5. Turn on both 50 psi gas sources.

6. Regulate air-oxygen concentration with front dial to desired percent.

Special Considerations

- Low flow module or special adjustments must be made on blenders to use for flows of gas less than 15 LPM.
- Many blenders have alarm systems to indicate when one source gas is low.
- Water trap should be used when compressor provides source of air.
- DISS standard fittings for air and oxygen on all blenders.

Hazards

- One gas source failure allowing use of the higher pressure gas source as the means of providing flow to the patient.

Maintenance

- Inlet filters should be checked periodically.
- Check oxygen concentrations with settings on blender to verify controls.

OXYGEN CONCENTRATOR

Description

This device extracts oxygen from room air and provides the patient with a continuous flow of oxygen enriched air.

Objective

To provide the patient with a source of oxygen-enriched air.
To limit the use of cylinders for the home oxygen therapy patient.

Procedure

1. Connect power line to grounded electrical source. Fill humidifier with sterile, distilled water.
2. Turn on power switch.
3. Adjust flow to desired level.
4. Check oxygen concentration on analyser. Adjust the flowmeter if necessary.
5. Connect oxygen administrating device to patient.
6. Adjust:

LPM	O_2%
2	94
4	88
6	72
8	62
10	53

Special Considerations

- Generally used for home use for those patients who use low-flow oxygen.
- Converts room air to 95% oxygen.
- May be noisy for the light sleeper.
- Most units available with oxygen analyser.
- Use humidifiers to prevent nasal mucosa irritation.
- Small cylinder backup should always be available.
- Alarms indicate low oxygen output or power failure.

Hazards

• Electrical line failure.
• Inadequate oxygen supply for patients who need high concentrations of oxygen at high-flow rates.

Maintenance

• Oxygen analyser fuel cell needs replacing periodically.
• Clean lint and dust filters PRN.
• Keep humidifier clean and filled with sterile, distilled water when in use.
• Use electrical line failure alarm in line.

BIBLIOGRAPHY

Brown, M., and Ziment, I.: Evaluation of an oxygen concentration in patients with COPD. Respir. Ther., *8*(5): 55, 1978.

Burton, G. G., Gee, G. N., and Hodgkin, J. G.: Respiratory Care, A Guide to Clinical Practice. Philadelphia, J. B. Lippincott Co., 1977.

Hunsinger, D., *et al.:* Respiratory Technology, A Procedure Manual. Reston, Va., Reston Publishing Co., 1973.

McPherson, S. P.: Respiratory Therapy Equipment. St. Louis, C. V. Mosby Co., 1977.

Young, J. A., and Crocker, D. (eds.): Principles and Practice of Respiratory Therapy (2nd ed.). Chicago, Year Book Publishers, 1976.

TECHNICAL INFORMATION

Air Products, Allentown, Penn. 18105
Puritan-Bennett Corp., Kansas City, Missouri 64106
Devilbiss, Somerset, Penn. 15501
Marx Medical, Inc., LaJolla, Cal. 92037
Bird Corporation, Palm Springs, Cal.
Hudson Oxygen Therapy Sales Co., Wadsworth, Ohio 44281

CHAPTER TWO

Humidity and Aerosol-Generating Devices

Diane Blodgett, R.R.T.

GENERAL CONSIDERATIONS FOR HUMIDITY AND AEROSOL GENERATORS

The therapeutic modalities that the respiratory care practitioner provides usually incorporate a humidifying and/or an aerosol-generating device. There are exceptions (*e.g.*, chest physiotherapy), but even these treatments may be preceded by aerosol or high humidity therapy.

The basic difference between humidifiers and aerosol generators is that a humidifying unit increases the water vapor content (molecular water) while aerosol generators create liquid suspended in a gas (particulate water).

The therapeutic objectives of humidity therapy are to humidify inspired gases and to prevent the loss of water vapor from the respiratory tract. The criteria for termination of humidity therapy are discontinuation of the inspiration of dry gases and the ability of the patient to maintain a neutral or slightly positive water balance.

The objectives of aerosol therapy are different because while humidity therapy prevents the loss of water, aerosol adds water to the respiratory system. The therapeutic objectives of aerosol therapy are to humidify inspired gases, hydrate the respiratory system, aid in the liquification of retained dry secretions, induce a cough to obtain a sputum specimen or promote bronchial hygiene, provide a method of delivering medication into the tracheobronchial tree and decrease laryngeal edema.

The criteria for termination of aerosol therapy are a normal fluid balance (0 humidity deficit), use of the normal anatomical humidification system (extubation), normal auscultatory sounds,

(Text continues on p. 44.)

Table 2-1. Humidifiers

Type	Examples	Humidity produced	Applications
Heated vaporizer	Hankscraft Devilbiss	100% RH at 21°C	Increases relative humidity of a small closed area.
Pass-over humidifier	Emerson Ventilator Bird Humidifier	100% RH at 37°C when heated	May be used for large bore tubing applications and/or ventilators, and high humidity for masks, tents, endotracheal tubes, etc.
Bubble diffuser (Simple humidifier)	Hudson Inspiron Bard Parker Ideal	40-50% RH at 21°C (room temperature) 20% RH at 37°C (body temperature)	For use with oxygen administering devices. *e.g.*, cannula, simple masks. Use where low humidity is adequate for patient's needs.
Bubble diffuser (Cascade humidifier)	Puritan Bennett Monaghan Respiratory Care, Inc.	100% RH at 21-37°C when heated	Can be used for any large bore tubing applications and/or ventilators, CPAP, high humidity with oxygen enrichment systems.

[41]

Table 2-2. Aerosol Generators

Type	Example	Aerosol/Output Characteristics	Applications
Atomizer a. Bulb b. Metered	a. Devilbiss b. Bronkometer Isuprel Mistometer	a/b. Wide range of particle sizes (30-100 μ) No baffle b. Amount of medication delivered varies, depending on manufacturer	Intermittent application of small amounts of medication.
Centrifugal–Spin disc	Devilbiss Hankscraft	Wide range of particle sizes and water vapor. 4-8ml./min. output	Room "Humidifier"—limited use.
Jet Nebulizer a. Large Volume	Puritan All Purpose Ohio Deluxe Microsonic Disposable (Bard Parker Inspiron)	1-40 μ range of particle size. 0.5-1ml./min. output 100% RH at BTPS	Humidify inspired gases. Continuous aerosol therapy.

b. Small Volume	Bird Mironebulizer Puritan Twin Jet Acorn Dantreband	1-40 μ range of particle size. 0.25-0.5ml./min. output	Humidify inspired gases. Intermittent aerosol therapy. Aerosolization of small amounts of medication.
Babbington	Solosphere Maxi-Cool Hydrosphere	3-5 μ range of particle size for 97% of aerosol produced 1-7ml./min. output 100% RH at BTFS	Continuous ⟩ Aerosol Intermittent ⟩ Therapy
Ultrasonic	Devilbiss Mistogen Monaghan Puritan Bennett	1-5 μ range of particle size. 1-6ml./min. output, depending on model. 100% RH at BTPS	Continuous ⟩ Aerosol Intermittent ⟩ Therapy

ability to mobilize secretions independently, relief of broncho-spasm, and relief of inspiratory stridor.

Each type of therapy may be given heated or unheated, and intermittently or continuously. Humidifiers are usually utilized on a continuous basis for gas administration and for mechanical ventilation. The advantages of humidifiers are that there is little chance of bacterial contamination and that the devices are simple to use and maintain. The disadvantage is the low relative humidity provided unless the unit is heated.

Aerosol generators are used on an intermittent basis to meet all of their previously mentioned therapeutic objectives, except humidification of dry gases and hydration of the respiratory system. In these instances, continuous aerosol is most appropriate. The advantages of aerosol generators are that they deposit a large amount of solution into both the upper and lower airways and that medications can be administered topically. Because of these advantages, the therapeutic objectives and goals of the therapy can be met. There are some disadvantages to the aerosol units. The aerosol itself can produce a reflex bronchospasm; it can provide a vehicle for bacteria transmission, and in some instances, it provides too much liquid into the cardio-respiratory system (overhydration).

Whatever the device chosen, the therapist should weigh the advantages and disadvantages of each method of therapy and choose that treatment modality which will accomplish the goal while providing the optimum level of patient care and safety. Evaluation of the patient, following the administration of the therapy, will help the therapist decide the appropriateness of the treatment being provided.

HEATERS FOR HUMIDIFIERS AND AEROSOL GENERATORS

Description

Aerosol humidifiers (or heaters) are designed to raise the temperature of the liquid in the reservoir. By increasing the temperature of the liquid, the relative humidity and output can be increased.

Objectives

To increase the relative humidity to 100% at body temperature. To decrease the humidity deficit.

Special Considerations

- Attach heated device to patient only after flow and temperature have stabilized.
- High temperature of solution may result in pulmonary burns.
- Do not use heater with small-bore tubing.
- Always monitor temperature of heated inspired gases.
- Watch tubing for water accumulation.
- Discard water accumulation. (Do not empty back into reservoir.)
- For heaters that are not adjustable, temperature of the inspired gas at the patient outlet may be increased or decreased by varying the tubing length. (Increase tubing length—decrease temperature; decrease tubing length—increase temperature.)
- Do not let the reservoir go dry.
- Heated aerosol or humidity may be uncomfortable to the patient who is breathing through his nose or mouth.
- Heated devices are generally used when the normal humidifying mechanism is by-passed (*i.e.*; endotracheal or tracheostomy tube in place).

Hazards

- Pulmonary burns.
- Overmobilization of secretions.
- Increased body temperature.

Maintenance

- Check electrical plugs for damage.
- Decontaminate immersion heaters following each use.
- Wipe surfaces of all other heaters with 1) mild cleansing agent, 2) rinse, 3) decontamination agent, and 4) rinse.

CHESTER COLLEGE LIBRARY

Table 2-3. Heaters for Humidifiers and Aerosol Generators

Type	Examples	Characteristics	Advantages	Disadvantages
Immersion (Fig. 2-1)	Puritan Inspiron	Rod-shaped electrical heater that extends into the jet nebulizer solution. Some models adjustable.	Simple to use. Relatively inexpensive. Solution visible.	Hot heater barrel—possible burns. Must use separate temperature monitoring and control system. Difficult to control temperature. Difficult to decontaminate. Difficult to service.
Wrap-around (Fig. 2-2)	Bard Parker	Wrap-around electric coil that encircles the jet nebulizer or humidifier jar.	Simple to use. Relatively inexpensive. No need to decontaminate.	May get hot to the touch. Impossible to see solution in reservoir. Cannot control heat. Must use separate temperature-monitoring and control system. Impossible to service.
Contact Pass-over (Fig. 2-3)	McGaw Ohio Chemetron Bird	Adjustable heater that attaches to base of jar or allows jet stream to come in contact with heater.	Adjustable control. No need to decontaminate, or element is part of nebulizer or humidifier. Solution visible.	Expensive. Must use separate temperature monitoring and control system. Must purchase custom jars to use with each type nebulizer (Ohio). McGaw only fits Solosphere. Chemetron and Bird cannot be interchanged with other units.

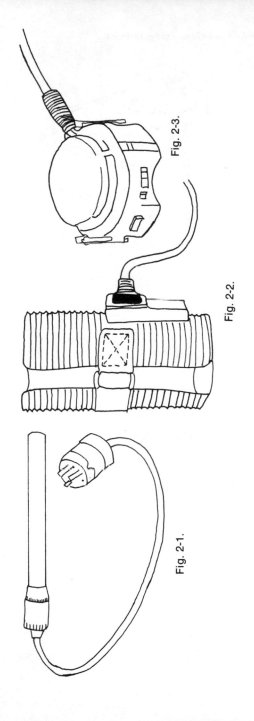

Fig. 2-3.

Fig. 2-2.

Fig. 2-1.

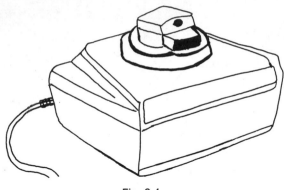

Fig. 2-4.

HEATED VAPORIZER

Description

Large heat-proof reservoir with immersion type heater. Water is drawn into heating column where steam (water vapor) is produced.

Objective

To increase the relative humidity in a small enclosed area (room), by producing water vapor (steam).

Procedure

1. Fill reservoir with tap water to fill-line.
2. Replace cover.
3. Place vaporizer about four feet from patient. Insert plug into electrical outlet.
4. Steam should be emitted from the vaporizer within 5-10 minutes.

Special Considerations

- Place vaporizer in safe position—the floor is best.
- Do not overfill.
- Use tap water-mineral content needed for proper operation.
- If steam is produced too slowly, unplug unit, add 0.25 ml. baking soda to water, mix well and plug unit in again.

- If steam is uneven or produced too rapidly, use half distilled water or clean unit thoroughly.
- Unplug unit before moving it.

Hazards

- Burns if not handled properly and with caution.
- Water damage if placed too close to walls.
- Shock if cord comes in contact with water.

Maintenance

- Clean after each use.
- Every five days, rinse unit with bleach and water.
- Remove mineral deposits with distilled white vinegar.

PASS-OVER HUMIDIFIER
(BIRD)

Description

This type of humidifier has a reservoir, a wick, housing inlet and outlet ports for tubing connection, and a heater.

Objective

To humidify inspired gases for either a high- or low-flow oxygen system by passing the gas near a heated wet wick.

Procedure

1. Before assembling the humidifier, it is necessary to insert a wick into the housing.
2. With the wick in place, replace the cap on the bottom of the housing.
3. Attach housing to controller. Replace cap on top of housing.
4. Place humidifier in line with patient.
5. Attach continuous water-feed system—float will maintain constant water level.
6. Make sure humidifier is plugged in.
7. Adjust the heater.
8. Turn on gas flow to warm delivery circuit.
9. Attach set-up to patient.

Special Considerations

- Continuous feed system.
- Low gas flow resistance.
- Fast warm-up time—less than 5 minutes.
- Monitor inspired gas temperature.
- Built-in high temperature alarm (visual and audible) shuts heater off at 41°C (105°F).
- A remote sensor monitors temperature at proximal airway.
- Provides 100% RH at 37°C.
- Adapts to use with ventilators, oxygen administration systems, tents.
- Can be used for humidification during neonatal ventilation because of low compliance factor (0.2ml./cm. H_2O).
- No smoking, flames or ungrounded electrical equipment in area of oxygen use.

Hazards

- Rain-out in tubing occluding the gas flow.
- Malfunction in humidifier controller.
- Minimal potential hazard for transmission of bacteria.

Maintenance

- Keep continuous water-feed system filled and open.
- Monitor temperature at patient wye.

BUBBLE-DIFFUSER HUMIDIFIER
(SIMPLE)

Description

This type of humidifier has a reservoir, a standard connection for a flowmeter, a diffuser made of a porous material and a small bore outlet connection.

Objective

To humidify inspired gases for low-flow oxygen system by diffusing the gas through water.

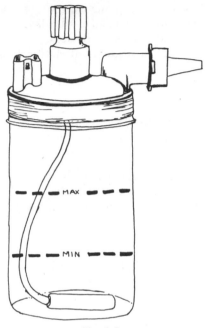

Fig. 2-5.

Procedure

1. Fill humidifier reservoir with sterile distilled water.
2. Replace top and attach humidifier to flowmeter.
3. Turn flow to 3 LPM to check for bubble production. Bubbles should be small and readily apparent.
4. Attach small bore tubing to humidifier. Connect oxygen-administering device to tubing.
5. Adjust flowmeter to appropriate setting.
6. Attach oxygen-administering device to patient.

Special Considerations

• Pop-off prevents excess pressure build-up when tubing kinks.
• Blockage of small bore outlet connection cuts off gas flow.
• Small chance of bacteria transfer with this type of unit.

- Provides 20% RH at 37°C to the patient.
- May be heated to increase relative humidity.
- Can only be used with low-flow devices.
- No smoking, flames or ungrounded electrical equipment in area of oxygen use.

Hazards

- Inadequate humidity for the patient's needs.

Maintenance

- Discard disposable units after use.
- Clean and decontaminate reusable units.
- Keep humidifier filled with sterile distilled water.

BUBBLE-DIFFUSER HUMIDIFIER
(CASCADE)

Description

This type of humidifier has a reservoir, a mesh diffuser, large bore inlet and outlet and usually an immersion heater.

Objective

To humidify inspired gases for a high-flow oxygen system by diffusing the gas through heated water.

Procedure

1. Fill humidifier reservoir with sterile distilled water.
2. Replace by screwing jar into cover.
3. Place the Cascade in line with patient.
4. Make sure Cascade is plugged in, if using heater assembly.
5. Adjust the heater.

Blue numbers 1-5—below body temperature ⎞
White numbers 6-7—body temperature   ⎬ On Bennett
Red numbers 8-9—above body temperature ⎠ Cascade I

6. Allow warm-up time.
7. Turn on gas flow to warm delivery circuit.
8. Attach set-up to patient.

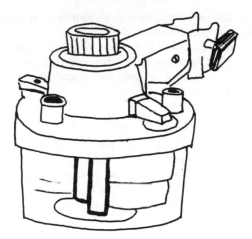

Fig. 2-6.

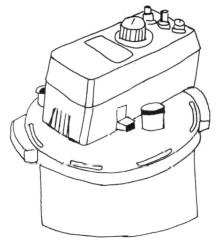

Fig. 2-7.

Special Considerations

- Use only sterile water to fill humidifier.
- Temperature of water vapor drops about 2°C per foot of tubing from humidifier.
- Can provide 100% RH at 37°C

- May be Servo-controlled (maintains and sets temperature).
- Warm-up time—15-20 minutes.
- High flow rates/fast ventilator rates = lower temperature.
- Low flow rates/slow ventilator rates = higher temperature.
- No smoking, flames or ungrounded electrical equipment in area of oxygen use.

Hazards

- Overheating causes pulmonary burns from dry, hot gas, if Cascade becomes dry.
- Minimal potential hazard for transmission of bacteria.
- Rain-out in tubing may occlude gas flow.
- Inadequate humidification for patient's need at unheated or low temperatures.

Maintenance

- Monitor temperature close to patient wye.
- Do not let fluid level fall below refill line.
- Check parts for wear (*i.e.,* especially rubber and silicone parts).
- Refill whenever necessary.

ATOMIZER—BULB

Description

Hand-held aerosol generator that uses the squeeze of a bulb to produce a flow of gas. The medication solution is drawn into the flow of gas and a mist is produced (30-100 μ range of particles).

Objective

To apply a medication locally into the upper airway, by generating an aerosol to be inhaled by the patient.

Procedure

1. Approach the patient and explain the procedure.
2. Remove the top of the atomizer and place medication solution into the reservoir.
3. Replace top.

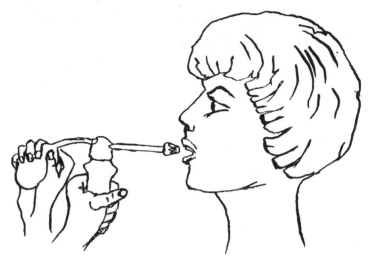

Fig. 2-8.

4. Have the patient open his mouth and breathe quietly.

5. Instruct the patient to inhale deeply and squeeze the bulb just after the initiation of inspiration.

6. Have the patient hold his breath 10-15 seconds and exhale slowly.

7. Repeat as directed.

Special Considerations

• Used mainly for applying medication to the upper airway.
• Difficult to control dosage.
• Wide range of particle sizes because a baffle is not incorporated.

Hazards

• Local irritation from medication. See specific medication hazards (Table 2-4).

Maintenance

• Clean atomizer following each use.

Table 2-4. Aerosol Medications

Medications	Examples	Dosage	Indications	Contraindications	Adverse Reactions
Bronchodilators	Isoetharine Isoproterenol Racemic Epinephrine	1% (0.25-1ml.) 1% (0.3ml.) } in saline 2.25% (0.25- 0.7ml.) } 3-4×day	Bronchial dilation Relief of bronchospasm	Hypersensitivity. Caution: Cardiac patients.	Tachycardia Nausea Palpitation Restlessness
	Atropine—derivatives (in research stage).	0.5-1%	Prevents or relieves bronchospasm.	Glaucoma Renal failure	Tachycardia Stiffens secretions
Decongestant	Phenolnephrine	0.25-1% (0.3-1ml.) in saline 3-4×day	Reduces edema Vasoconstriction	Hypersensitivity. Display of "rebound" effect.	Elevated systolic and diastolic
Antiobiotics	Carbenicillin	10-20 mg. in saline 3×day	Gram-negative bacteria (Pseudomonas)	These drugs are of questionable value for use by inhalation. Oral routes should be utilized where appropriate.	Bronchospasm Hypersensitivity
	Kanamycin	50-400 mg. in saline 3×day	Gram-negative bacteria (Proteus)		
	Neomycin	50-400 mg. in saline 2-4×day	Gram-negative bacteria (Staphylococcus/ Haemophilus)		
	Polymyxin B	10-50 mg. in saline 3-4×day	Gram-negative bacteria (Pseudomonas)		

	Amphotericin B	5-20 mg. in saline 2-4×day	Fungal infections (aspergillosis, histoplasmosis)		Bronchospasm. Decomposes rubber and metal equipment.
Mucolytics	Acetylcysteine	10% recommended undiluted. 20% Dilute 1-1 with H_2O or normal saline	To break up mucus	Asthmatic patients receiving aerosolized penicillin Hypersensitivity to preparation.	
	Ethyl alcohol	20-50%	Pulmonary edema	Alcoholics	Irritation of lung tissue.
	H_2O	—	Aids in the liquefaction and mobilization of secretions		Usually well tolerated.
	$NaHCO_3$	4-7%			
	NaCl	0.45-0.9%-15%	Vehicle for medication delivery.	High saline conc. for use in cardiac patients.	Sodium retention of fluids.
Proteolytics	Pancreatic dornase	100,000 units in saline 2-3×day	Purulent secretions.	Other mucolytics may be just as effective.	Bronchospasm.
Steroids	Hydrocortisone	5-30 mg./day	Control of asthma attacks.	In treatment of status asthmaticus and acute episodes of asthma.	Adrenal suppression.

(Continued on overleaf)

Table 2-4. Aerosol Medications (Continued)

Medications	Examples	Dosage	Indications	Contraindications	Adverse Reactions
Steroids *(Cont.)*				Hypersensitivity to preparation.	
	Dexamethasone	1mg./day			
	Triamcinolone (unavailable to us)	0.8-2mg./day metered dose			Suppression of HPA function.
	Beclomethosone (drug of choice)	1-3mg./day metered dose			*Candida* infections in throat.
Antiasthmatic	Cromolyn sodium	80mg./day using a spinhaler	Prevent asthma attack.	Hypersensitivity to preparation.	Hoarseness. Upper airway irritation. Bronchospasm Coughing

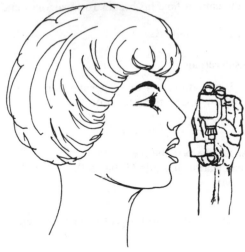

Fig. 2-9.

ATOMIZER—METERED DOSE

Description

Hand-held aerosol generator that uses a pressurized canister to force the medication through a small jet. Mouthpiece directs flow to patient.

Objective

To deliver a metered aerosol dosage of a medication to the patient.

Procedure

1. Approach the patient and explain the procedure.
2. Attach the mouthpiece to the medication canister.
3. Direct the patient to place his index finger on top of the canister and his thumb at the bottom of the mouthpiece.
4. Instruct the patient to hold the mouthpiece about 2 inches from his mouth and inhale deeply. Just after the initiation of inspiration, have the patient compress the mouthpiece and canister.

5. Have the patient hold his breath 10-15 seconds and exhale slowly.

6. Repeat as directed.

Special Considerations

• Usually 2-3 inhalations 3-4 times per day for most bronchodilators. Follow instructions for physician.

Hazards

• Over-dosages are possible.
• Specific medication hazards (Table 2-4).

Maintenance

• Clean mouthpiece daily to prevent clogging of jet.

BEDSIDE HUMIDIFIER
(SPIN-DISC NEBULIZER)

Description

Large water reservoir with a spinning disc that draws water up and propels it against a grate to produce a fine mist.

Objective

To increase the relative humidity in a small enclosed area (room) by producing a mist which evaporates.

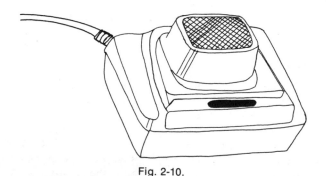

Fig. 2-10.

Procedure

1. Fill reservoir with distilled water. Replace lid.
2. Place humidifier on flat surface, close to the patient.
3. Insert plug into electrical outlet.
4. Turn on switch.

Special Considerations

- Do not over fill.
- Use distilled water.
- To protect surface underneath humidifier, place unit on tray.
- Do not add medication to the water.
- Humidifier *can* run dry—it will recirculate the air.

Hazards

- Shock, if cord comes in contact with water.
- Water damage, if placed too close to walls.
- Bacterial contamination.

Maintenance

- Clean filters daily.
- Clean after each use with soap and water.
- Never submerge cover.
- Rinse unit with bleach and water (every five days).
- Remove mineral deposits with distilled white vinegar.

JET NEBULIZER—LARGE VOLUME

Description

Jet nebulizer is an atomizer with a baffle, which produces an aerosol that has a stable range of particle size (less than 30 μ). A large jet nebulizer has a reservoir, a gas inlet and outlet, jet syphon tube, and a system of baffles.

Objective

To provide continuous output of aerosol (heated or unheated) and to humidify inspired gases (heated or unheated).

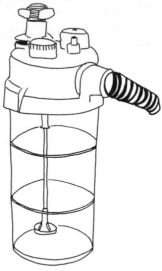

Fig. 2-11.

Procedure

1. Approach the patient and explain the procedure.
2. Fill the nebulizer with sterile distilled water to the fill-line.
3. Attach nebulizer to flowmeter.
4. Adjust flow to 12 LPM to check for aerosol production. ($F_{I_{O_2}}$ will depend on source gas and nebulizer entrainment setting.)
5. Attach large bore tubing to nebulizer.
6. Connect aerosol-administering device to end of large bore tubing.
7. Set selection dial for oxygen concentration.
8. Attach device to patient and adjust flow to keep mist visible.

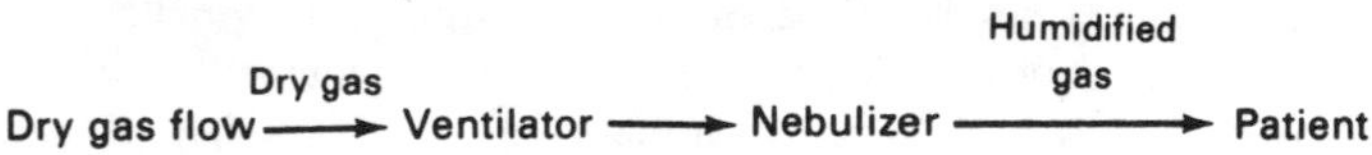

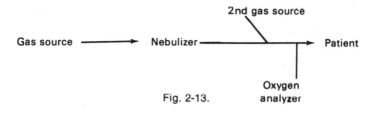

Fig. 2-12

Oxygen Concentration can be varied.

1. Use Blender with 100% Source Gas.
2. Air Gas source with oxygen bled in (low concentration).
3. Oxygen Gas source with air bled in (high concentration).

Fig. 2-13.

Increase Flow can be provided by running two nebulizers into wye.

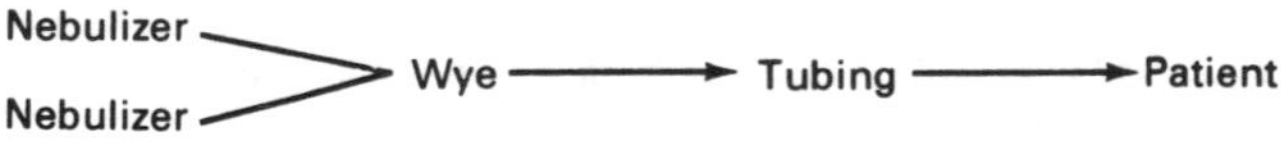

Fig. 2-14.

Special Considerations

- Safety relief valve to vent excessive build-up of pressure.
- Dilution control—entrains air for desired oxygen concentration.
- May be used heated or unheated.
- Most units should be used only with large bore tubing. (Puritan

All-Purpose can be used on 100% setting with small bore tubing. Do not use heated with small bore tubing.)
- Keep jar filled. Do not let unit run dry.
- When water condenses in tubing, drain and discard.
- When using a T-tube, add reservoir tubing to expiration side of T-tube to stabilize oxygen concentration to the patient.
- Monitor F_{IO_2} when oxygen is used as source gas.
- May be used in line with ventilation devices to provide humidification of inspired gases. (Fig. 2-12)
- Oxygen concentration can be varied (Fig. 2-13)
- To increase flow, see Figure 2-14.
- May be used on intermittent basis—there are units that produce a better output and range of particle size which is more appropriate for intermittent use (See Ultrasonic and Babington Nebulizers).
- No smoking, flames or ungrounded electrical equipment in area of oxygen use.

$$F_{IO_2} = \frac{O_2 \text{ flow in LPM} + (0.21) \text{ Air Flow in LPM}}{\text{Total Flow}}$$

Hazards

- Pulmonary burns with heated unit that overheats or runs dry.
- Water accumulation can block gas flow to patient.
- Drying of mucosa when nebulizer runs dry.
- Bacterial contamination and transmission.

Maintenance

- Replace unit every 24 hours.
- Decontaminate or sterilize after each use.
- Replace worn parts.
- Empty unit before refilling. Rinse and fill with sterile water.

JET NEBULIZER—SMALL VOLUME

Description

The small volume jet nebulizer produces an aerosol that has a stable range of particle size (less than 30 μ). It has a small reservoir (less than 20 ml.), a gas inlet and outlet, jet syphon tube and a baffle system.

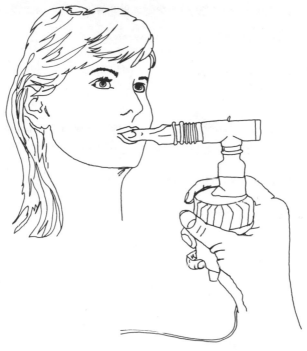

Fig. 2-15.

Objective

To deliver small amounts of medication to the patient and to humidify inspired gases.

Procedure

1. Approach the patient and explain the procedure.
2. Attach the nebulizer to the source gas.
3. Fill the nebulizer with the medication prescribed.
4. Turn on the gas flow and adjust flow to nebulizer so that a fine mist is visible.
5. Auscultate the chest and monitor vital signs.
6. Instruct the patient to breathe deeply and hold his breath briefly at the end of inspiration. He should exhale slowly.
7. Instruct the patient to breathe deeply again, and cough.

Source gas can be provided in a variety of ways.

    a. Primary gas source is air or oxygen.

    b. Air ———→ into wye

        Oxygen

                               Small bore tubing into

    c. Blender with low flow module.   nebulizer ———→ Patient

    d. IPPB

    e. Ventilator

Fig. 2-16.

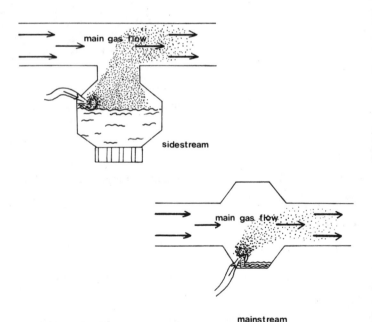

sidestream

mainstream

Fig. 2-17. Nebulizer used as sidestream or mainstream. (Modified from: McPherson, S.: Respiratory Therapy Equipment. St. Louis, C. V. Mosby Co., 1977.)

8. Continue therapy for 10-15 minutes or until medication is nebulized. Monitor vital signs and breath sounds.

9. At the completion of the therapy, evaluate the patient for changes in vital signs and breath sounds. Note sputum production and characteristics.

10. Empty nebulizer and rinse. Rinse and dry patient appliance.

Special Considerations

- Source gas can be provided in a variety of ways. (Fig. 2-16)
- Must use small bore tubing to power small jet nebulizer.
- Nebulizer may be used as mainstream or sidestream nebulizer. (Fig. 2-17)
- Monitor vital signs, breath sounds and sputum production before treatment, and during and following therapy.
- Nebulizer may be permanent or disposable.
- No smoking, sparks, flames, or ungrounded electrical equipment in area when oxygen is used as source gas.

Hazards

- Bacterial contamination.
- Side effects of medications delivered.

Maintenance

- Exchange nebulizer, tubing and patient appliance every 24 hours.
- Decontaminate or sterilize after each use.
- Keep the jet clean to maximize output.
- Replace worn parts.

ULTRASONIC NEBULIZERS

Description

A solution contained in a chamber is vibrated at a high rate, producing a geyser that breaks the solution into very small particles. A flow of gas carries the particles to the patient. This unit has a power source, couplant chamber, nebulizer chamber, and gas flow inlet and outlet.

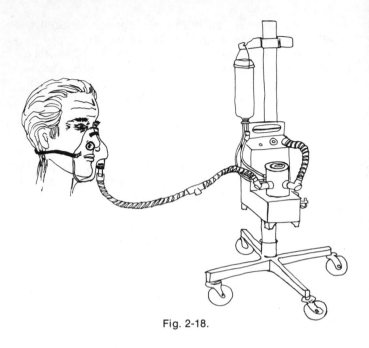

Fig. 2-18.

Objective

To produce an aerosol with small, stable particle size (1-8 μ) to be used intermittently or continuously for aerosol therapy.

Procedure

Intermittent Use

1. Approach the patient and explain the procedure.
2. Place the ultrasonic unit on level surface or use a stand.
3. Plug cord into electrical outlet.
4. Fill couplant chamber with tap water to fill-line.
5. Place nebulizer chamber into couplant chamber and secure it.
6. Fill nebulizer chamber to fill-line with sterile solution to be nebulized.
7. Connect nebulizer chamber to gas flow outlet.
8. Attach large-bore tubing to outlet of nebulizer chamber.
9. Connect other end of large-bore tubing to patient appliance (*i.e.,* aerosol mask, T-tube).
10. Auscultate the chest and monitor vital signs.

11. Place appliance on patient and instruct him to breathe through his mouth.

12. Instruct patient to breathe deeply every few breaths, hold briefly at the end of inspiration, and exhale slowly.

13. Increase output of ultrasonic to level that is easily tolerated by patient.

14. Have the patient breathe deeply and cough.

15. Continue therapy for 10-15 minutes. Monitor vital signs and breath sounds.

16. At the completion of the therapy, evaluate the patient for changes in vital signs and breath sounds. Note sputum production and characteristics.

17. Empty nebulizer chamber and rinse. Rinse and dry patient appliance.

Continuous Use

1. Approach the patient and explain the procedure.

2. Place the ultrasonic unit on level surface or use a stand.

3. Plug cord into electrical outlet.

4. Fill sterile supply bottle with desired sterile solution (half-normal saline is recommended).

5. Connect feed system to supply bottle.

6. Fill couplant chamber with tap water to fill-line.

7. Place nebulizer chamber in couplant chamber.

8. Attach feed system to nebulizer chamber and allow solution to fill chamber.

9. Attach nebulizer chamber to gas flow outlet.

10. Attach large-bore tubing to outlet of nebulizer chamber.

11. Connect the large-bore tubing to the patient appliance (face tent, aerosol mask, croupette, mist tent).

12. Turn on generator and adjust to desired level (flush initially for a tent).

13. Position appliance on patient.

14. Evaluate the therapy: monitor vital signs, breath sounds and sputum production initially, and every four hours and PRN.

Special Considerations

Output
Devilbiss 65-0-6ml./min.
35B-0-3ml./min.
900-0-3ml./min.
800-0-6ml./min.

Monaghan   650-0-3ml./min.
            670-0-3ml./min.
            675-0-6ml./min.
Mistogen   142/143-0-3ml./min.
            145-0-6ml./min.

- May be used in line with ventilation devices to provide humidification of inspired gases (Fig. 2-19).
- Monitor F_{IO_2} when using oxygen as source gas.
- Monitor vital signs, breath sounds and sputum production before treatment, and during and following therapy.
- Have suction equipment on hand to clear secretions, if necessary.
- For patients who develop bronchospasm, bronchodilator administration before the therapy may be appropriate.
- Daily weights should be obtained on infants and small children receiving continuous ultrasonic therapy.
- Disposable nebulizer chambers are available; some are prefilled.
- Most ultrasonics have an optional drug vial to administer small amounts of medication.
- No smoking, sparks, flames or ungrounded electrical equipment in area when oxygen is used as source gas.

Hazards

- Reflex bronchospasm.
- Bacterial contamination.
- Fluid overload in infants and small children.
- Shocks.
- Overmobilization of secretions.
- Water accumulation can block gas flow to patient.
- Specific medication hazards (Table 2-4).

Use large-bore tubing from nebulizer chamber to patient.

Source gas from:

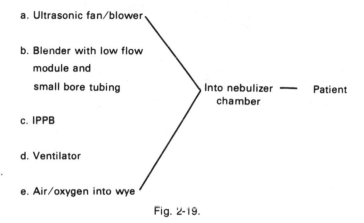

a. Ultrasonic fan/blower

b. Blender with low flow
module and
small bore tubing

Into nebulizer —— Patient
chamber

c. IPPB

d. Ventilator

e. Air/oxygen into wye

Fig. 2-19.

Maintenance

- Check tubing frequently to prevent obstruction in tubing by water accumulation.
- For continuous use, keep reservoir liquid above fill-line to insure that nebulizer chamber does not run dry.
- Exchange nebulizer chamber, large-bore tubing and patient appliance.
- Clean filters between patients and when necessary.

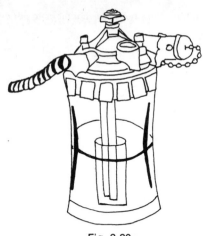

Fig. 2-20.

BABINGTON NEBULIZER

Description

These devices use the hydronamic principle to produce an aerosol that has a stable particle size and high output. These units contain a reservoir, aerosol generator, gas inlet and outlet, venturi and filter(s).

Objective

To humidify inspired gases and to provide a continuous or intermittent output of aerosol.

Procedure

See large volume nebulizer procedure.
See ultrasonic nebulizer procedure.

Special Considerations

- Maxi-Cool ⎫ up to 7ml./min. output—will drop temperature
- Hydrosphere ⎭ 6-10°F below ambient.
- Solosphere—2ml./min. output—can be heated.
- Monitor F_{IO_2} when oxygen is source gas.

- Monitor vital signs, breath sounds and sputum production, before therapy, and during and following therapy.
- Use as a continuous aerosol such as jet nebulizer (Solosphere) or as ultrasonic nebulizer, either on an intermittent or continuous basis.
- No smoking, sparks, flames or ungrounded electrical equipment when oxygen is used as source gas.

Hazards

- Reflex bronchospasm
- Fluid overload
- Overmobilization of secretions
- Bacterial Contamination.
- Water accumulation can block gas flow to patient.

Maintenance

- Check tubing frequently to prevent obstruction in the tubing by water accumulation.
- To insure that nebulizer chamber does not run dry in continuous use, keep reservoir liquid above fill-line.
- If unit stops misting, lift nebulizer chamber top to eliminate vapor lock. Replace top and unit should start to mist.
- Exchange nebulizer chamber, large-bore tubing and patient appliance every 24 hours.
- Clean filters daily.

BIBLIOGRAPHY

Burton, G. G., Gee, G. N., and Hodgkin, J. G.: Respiratory Care, A Guide to Clinical Practice. Philadelphia, J. B. Lippincott Company, 1977.

DeKornfeld, T.: Pharmacology for Respiratory Therapy. Sarasota, Glenn Educational Medical Services, Inc., 1976.

Egan, D.: Fundamentals of Respiratory Therapy. St. Louis, C. V. Mosby Co., 1977.

McPherson, S.: Respiratory Therapy Equipment. St. Louis, C. V. Mosby Co., 1977.

Mathewson, H. S.: Pharmacology for Respiratory Therapists. St. Louis, C. V. Mosby Co., 1977.

Rau, J., and Rau, M.: Fundamental Respiratory Therapy Equipment: Principles of Use and Operation. Sarasota, Glenn Educational Medical Services, Inc., 1977.

Shapiro, B., Morrison, R., Trout, C.: Clinical Applications of Respiratory Care. Chicago, Yearbook Medical Publishers, 1975.
Young, J.: Principles and Practice of Respiratory Therapy. Chicago, Yearbook Medical Publishers, Inc., 1976.

TECHNICAL INFORMATION

Hospal (Monaghan), Littleton, Colorado
Devilbiss, Somerset, Pennsylvania
Puritan Bennett, Kansas City, Missouri
McGaw, Irvine, California
Bird, Palm Springs, California
Ohio, Madison, Wisconsin
Chemetron, St. Louis, Missouri
Bard Parker, Rutherford, New Jersey
Inspiron, Upland, California
Mistogen, Oakland, California
Bendix, Davenport, Iowa

CHAPTER THREE

Hyperinflation Therapy

Terry Houts, B.S. R.R.T.

GENERAL CONSIDERATIONS FOR HYPERINFLATION THERAPY

The prevention or treatment of atelectasis is one of the respiratory therapist's primary concerns. In this section we will examine therapeutic modalities which encourage hyperinflation of the lung. Included in the section are rebreathing devices, incentive spirometry, and intermittent positive pressure breathing procedures. Other forms of therapy which encourage hyperinflation, e.g., CO_2/O_2 mixtures and breathing exercises, are covered in the chapters on Gas Administration and Chest Physiotherapy.

The primary therapeutic objectives of hyperinflation therapy are the prevention of atelectasis in the post-operative or sedentary patient, and the treatment of atelectasis by encouragement of deep inspiration. The development of atelectasis is a risk for patients undergoing thoracic, upper abdominal, or orthopaedic procedures requiring immobilization, and hyperinflation therapy may benefit them. It may also improve the clearance of secretions from the airways, and aid in the delivery of aerosolized medications.

The following are general considerations for each generic category of hyperinflation devices.

A. Rebreathing tubes or canisters are employed to increase the patient's anatomical dead space. This increase in space causes the patient to rebreathe a portion of his exhaled gases. This, in turn, increases the partial pressure of carbon dioxide contained in the lungs and arterial blood. The response of the body to increased amounts of carbon dioxide in the inspired air varies from individual to individual and even in the same person at different times. Both the central and peripheral chemo-receptors are sensitive to changes in the carbon dioxide tension of the blood. Each set of receptors reacts and triggers an increase in both the depth and rate of ventilation. Due to the varying responses to rebreathing devices, it is essential to monitor the patient closely. Values as high as 10-20% carbon dioxide may be reached with a rebreathing device. Use of this device is contraindicated for those patients who are physically unable to increase their tidal and minute ventilation in response to the carbon dioxide. For these patients an acute elevation of the arterial carbon dioxide tension and attendent side effects may result.

B. Incentive spirometers represent the second major category of hyperinflation devices. These units are used to encourage the patient to take a maximal sustained inspiration. The process of incentive spirometry emphasizes the inspiratory phase of the respiratory cycle. Incentive spirometry encourages the patient to inhale to maximum capacity. The basic goal of incentive spirometry is the prevention of atelectasis by exercising the patient's lung fields. Deep breathing helps to prevent the collapse of alveoli, to re-expand atelectatic areas of the lung and to stimulate the cough mechanism. Incentive spirometers provide a visual stimulus to encourage the patient, as well as a mechanical means by which the therapist and physician may monitor the patient's progress. The patient using this device should be visited often, encouraged to perform the maneuvers on his own, and have his progress, or lack thereof, monitored. There are minimal hazards with this device, although hyperventilation is possible with an over-zealous performer. (See detailed procedures.) The only contraindication to its use is the uncooperative patient.

C. Intermittent positive pressure breathing (IPPB) represents the third general category of hyperinflation therapy. IPPB involves the administration to the airway of gas under positive pressure, as a means of increasing the inspired volume. Since the majority of devices used for IPPB are pressure-limited, the volume exhaled should be monitored to assure an increase in tidal volume. Most IPPB machines have a nebulizer which allows the simultaneous administration of pharmacologic agents. Supplemental oxygen may also be administered during the IPPB treatment.

IPPB therapy is primarily indicated for those patients who are unable to increase spontaneously their tidal volume and/or are having trouble mobilizing their secretions. In patients with obstructive lung disease, it should be used with caution to prevent an increase in air trapping and possible pneumothorax when the patient coughs. The only absolute contraindication to IPPB is untreated tension pneumothorax. Hazards include hypo- and hyperventilation, decreased cardiac output and pneumothorax. (See detailed procedure.) IPPB may be discontinued when the patient exhibits the ability to increase spontaneously his tidal volume and cough effectively.

Regardless of the hyperinflation therapy employed it is important to quantify the amount of inflation achieved. Assessment of the overall effectiveness of the therapy must include a comparison of the volume of air exchanged during the therapy to the patient's normal spontaneous ventilation. Unless a significant increase in volume is achieved, the hyperinflation therapy may be of questionable benefit. In order to assess the need for continued therapy effectively, the patient's total ability in terms of sensorium, muscle strength, caloric intake, etc., must be considered in reference to his respiratory function. The criterium for termination is the ability of the patient to maintain the integrity of his respiratory function. This is ascertained through the evaluation of voluntary lung volumes and flow mechanics, the ending of acute post-op period, and obtaining a clear chest X-ray and normal auscultatory sounds.

REBREATHING DEVICES

Description

A rebreathing device consists of a cylindrical tube or canister, of approximately one liter in volume. It has a mouthpiece at one end and may provide an inlet for a supplemental oxygen flow.

Objectives

To increase mechanical deadspace, Pa_{CO_2}, tidal volume and minute ventilation, and to induce a deep inspiratory maneuver.

Procedure

1. Approach the patient and explain the procedure.
2. Place patient in semi-Fowlers or sitting position when possible.
3. Place nose clip snugly on patient's nostrils.

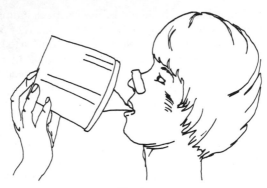

Fig. 3-1.

4. Have patient breathe *normally* both into and out through the device.

5. After five minutes *or* when the patient's tidal or minute volume has doubled discontinue the therapy.

6. Monitor patient until rate and/or volume approach normal resting values.

Special Considerations

- These devices should not be used in patients who, due to weakness or disability, cannot increase their ventilation voluntarily.
- Patient's pulse, respirations, and sensorium must be closely monitored during therapy.
- It is recommended that the depth and rate of respiration be monitored with a spirometer.
- Oxygen or aerosol therapy may be administered during the therapy by entraining aerosol-oxygen mixtures through the device. Devices which provide a continuous flow through the unit are unacceptable.

Hazards

- Carbon dioxide narcosis in individuals with chronic respiratory disease, hypercapnia, tachycardia, agitation, cardiac arrhythmia, hypertension, or increased intracranial pressure.

Maintenance

- The rebreathing device should be changed daily to reduce the risk of infection.

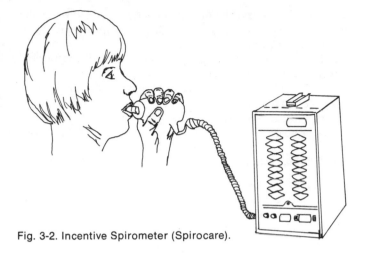

Fig. 3-2. Incentive Spirometer (Spirocare).

INCENTIVE SPIROMETRY

Description

The incentive spirometer is a device which provides visual reinforcement to encourage the patient to make a maximal inspiratory effort. The device provides the patient and therapist a means of monitoring progress toward a normal or predetermined goal.

Objective

To encourage patients to take intermittent spontaneous maximal inspirations to prevent or reverse atelectasis, shunting, hypoxia, and hypercarbia.

To aid in the removal of ascitis in the postop LeVeen Shunt patient.

Procedure

1. Approach the patient and explain the procedure.
2. Place the unit in a location convenient for the patient to see and use.
3. Position the patient in an erect, sitting or semi-Fowlers position whenever possible.
4. Have the patient place the mouthpiece in his mouth and inhale slowly, maintaining a constant flow through the unit. When the patient reaches maximal inspiration he should hold his breath for two to three seconds, and then exhale slowly.

5. Following the exhalation, encourage the patient to breathe normally for a short period of time. This will help prevent hyperventilation and tiring of the patient.

6. Have the patient repeat the maneuver until the desired number of goals is achieved.

7. The patient should be encouraged and coached in coughing during the treatment.

8. As patient tolerance grows, increase the volume and number of goals.

Special Considerations

- Aid the patient by splinting incisions.
- Preoperative instruction, including demonstration of diaphragmatic breathing, is desirable for those patients who are likely candidates for postoperative therapy.
- Determination of preoperative capacity aids in determining postoperative goals.
- Unit must be located in an area where it is readily accessible to the patient and the patient encouraged to use it between regular treatment times.
- Patients who are unable to initiate a significant inspiratory effort spontaneously are not good candidates for incentive spirometry.
- Use resistance in line for the LeVeen Shunt patient. The patient should inhale against a resistance.

Hazards

- Hyperventilation and related side effects.

INCENTIVE SPIROMETERS

Flow-Displaying Devices

Description

Lightweight units which incorporate an easily visualized indicator inside a flow tube to indicate patient's inspiratory effort.

Considerations for Use

Since the primary goal of incentive spirometry is to have the patient increase his *tidal volume* (T.V.), patients using these

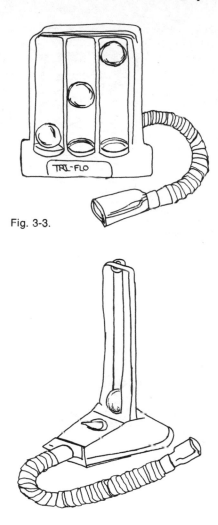

Fig. 3-3.

Fig. 3-4.

devices must be encouraged to suspend the indicator in the flow tube at a determined level for as long a period of time as possible. Many of these units make provision for administering aerosols. The flow from the aerosol generator may have to be added to the patient's inspired flow in order to estimate true volumes achieved by the patient. The flow-registering tube must be maintained in an upright position in order to indicate patient effort accurately.

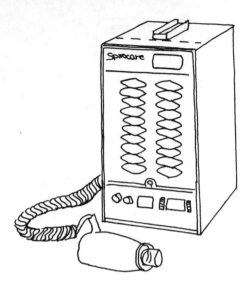

Fig. 3-5.

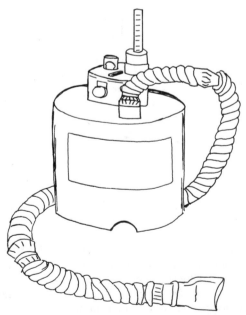

Fig. 3-6.

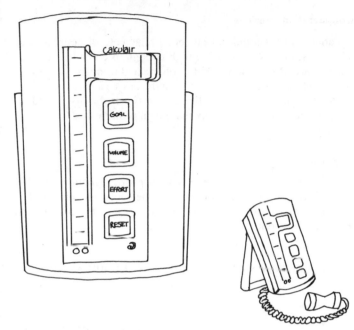

Fig. 3-7. Incentive Spirometer (Calculair).

Maintenance

Units are designed for use by a single patient and re-sterilization is generally not recommended. Units should be checked for free and uniform movement of the flow indicator before use.

Volume-Displaying Devices

Description

Units have two basic categories: flow sensing volume display unit, and volume displacement units. The flow-sensing volume display units utilize a flow-registering mouthpiece which is connected to a volume display panel. These units require an electrical or battery source, and record patient goals as well as volume. The volume displacement units consist of a piston or bellows contained in a housing. Calibrated indicators display the inspiratory volume achieved by the patient.

Considerations for Use

Patient goals should not be set so high as to discourage use. The goals, however, must be high enough to constitute a challenge. Careful selection of both volume and frequency is essential in encouraging the patient to use the device in between visits by the therapist. Patients utilizing both types of units should be encouraged to hold their maximal inspiration for a short period of time.

Maintenance

Units must be checked regularly for proper function and display. Batteries and light bulbs must be replaced periodically. Current leakage must be monitored in those units operating on alternating current.

INTERMITTENT POSITIVE PRESSURE BREATHING (IPPB)

Description

IPPB is the application of a positive inspiratory pressure, followed by a passive exhalation through the use of a volume-, flow-, or pressure-generating device.

Objectives

To provide a mechanical means of increasing tidal and/or minute alveolar ventilation, to aid in the prevention and treatment of atelectasis, hypercapnia and hypoxemia, to reduce temporarily the work of breathing, and to aid in the administration of aerosolized medicaments.

Procedures

1. Approach patient and explain the procedure.
2. Position the patient in an upright, sitting or semi-Fowlers position if possible.
3. Assemble therapy unit and check for proper function.
4. Add medicament to nebulizer, check for proper function. Nebulizer flow should be adequate but not excessive.
5. Determine patient's spontaneous tidal volume or vital capacity, pulse and respiration rate; auscultate chest.

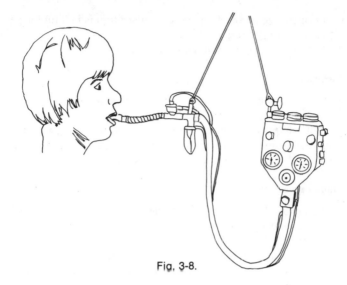

Fig. 3-8.

6. If controls are provided, adjust sensitivity to −1 or −2 cm.H_2O level.

7. If using mouthpiece, place nose clips on patient's nostrils.

8. Initiate treatment using moderate pressures, approximately 15 cmwp.

9. Increase pressure and adjust peak-flow controls (if provided) to obtain optimum pressure/flow pattern required to achieve desired tidal volume (10-15 ml./kg.).

10. Continue to monitor exhaled tidal volumes during treatment.

11. Continue treatment for specified period of time or until the prescribed medication is delivered.

12. Encourage the patient to cough.

13. Supporting incisions may be required.

Special Considerations

- An airtight connection between the machine and the patient's airway must be maintained. A variety of devices may be utilized for this purpose (See accessories).
- Exhaled volumes should be monitored to assure that the therapeutic goal is achieved.

- Pre-operative instruction and demonstration is helpful for patients who may require the therapy.
- Monitor vital signs throughout therapy.

Hazards

- IPPB is contraindicated in untreated pneumothorax.
- Hazards associated with IPPB include hemoptysis, hypoventilation, hyperventilation, pneumothorax, over-oxygenation, increased intrathoracic pressure with decreased cardiac output, and increased intracranial pressure.

Maintenance

- The entire IPPB device should be serviced and calibrated at regular intervals.
- Routine sterilization of the unit may be desirable although not absolutely required with the use of proper bacterial filters.
- The patient set-up should be either cleaned or sterilized after each use.

IPPB DEVICES

Electrically powered, manually cycled devices (e.g., Bird Asmastik Bennett TO and TA Series, Ohio Hand-E-Vent, etc.)

Description

Compact, lightweight units which employ a compressor fitted with a pressure unit (25-30 cm.H_2O) and connected to a nebulizer–exhalation valve–mouthpiece assembly. Breathing frequency, airway pressure, and tidal volume are determined by the patient's closing andopening the exhalation valve.

Considerations for Use

The units are specifically designed for home use and do not offer the flow/pressure capabilities generally required for intensive therapy. Since the patient controls the inspiratory time and therefore tidal volume, it is essential that thorough instruction and coaching be given in the proper technique for increasing tidal volume. Most units employ a venturi to increase the total flow through the units. As back pressure increases, the flow from the

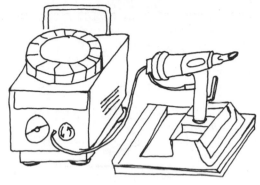

Fig. 3-9.

machine slows. Patients who breathe ''against'' the machine and not with it will receive smaller tidal volumes during the same inspiratory time.

Electrically powered, patient-sensing units (*e.g.*, Bird Portabird, Bennett AP series, Monaghan 505, 515)

Description

Self-contained units consisting of a compressor, an internal pressure regulator and patient-sensitive valve for beginning and ending inspiration. These units are fitted with an external patient supply tube, nebulizer and exhalation valve.

Considerations for Use

These units combine the portability and ease of operation required for home therapy with the convenience of a patient-assisting or sensing valve. The units may have a either pre-set or an adjustable limit for pressures achieved, as well as for the effort required to cycle the machine into inspiration. Several of these units also incorporate inspiratory flow rate controls, used to vary the flow of gas to the patient. Provision is also made to regulate the rate of nebulization. In setting the nebulization control, care must be exercised to prevent diversion of too much of the compressor's output to the nebulizer, decreasing the main flow of gas to the patient.

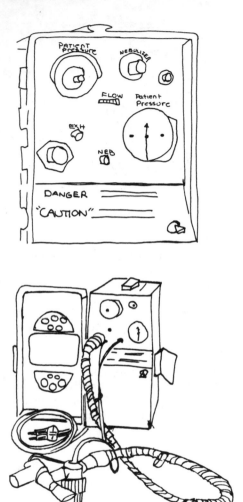

Fig. 3-10. IPPB (Monaghan 515).

Pneumatically powered patient-sensing devices (*e.g.*, Bird Mark 7 & 8, Bennett PR, TV, PV series, Monaghan 505 & 520)

Description

These units are powered by a 50 p.s.i. compressed gas source. Units may be cycled into inspiration either by patient effort or by a preset timing device. Inspiration is generally terminated by

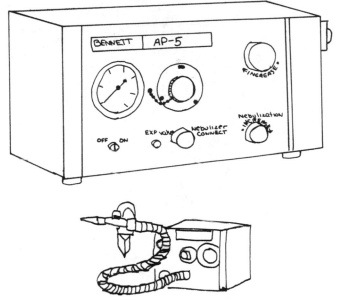

Fig. 3-11. IPPB (AP-5).

achieving a preset pressure, although flow or time may also be a basis for limiting inspiration. Most units provide controls which allow the direct adjustment of inspiratory flow rates. Nebulization is provided through a parallel flow system which, due to the source gas pressure available, does not effect the mainflow of gas to the patient.

Considerations for Use

These units are most commonly used in the hospital setting where a standard 50 p.s.i. source of oxygen or air is readily available. The units, when properly applied, can increase tidal volumes even in the face of very poor compliance or high resistance. By adjusting the pressure required and/or the flow rate of the delivered gas, a maximal increase in ventilation with minimal application of positive pressure may be achieved. In order to achieve this goal it is necessary to titrate pressure and flow rates to each individual patient carefully.

Various accessories are available to administer therapy.

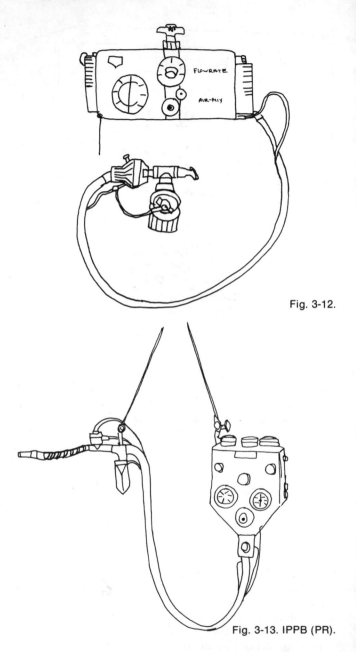

Fig. 3-12.

Fig. 3-13. IPPB (PR).

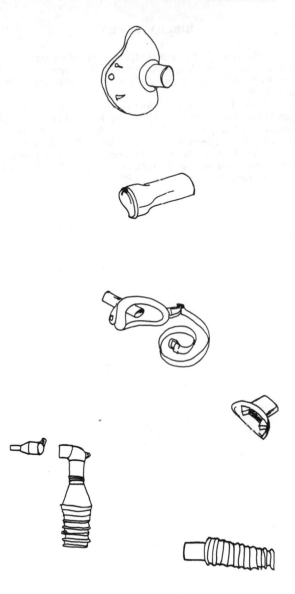

Fig. 3-14. IPPB (Accessories).

BIBLIOGRAPHY

Burton, G. G., Gee, G. N., and Hodgkin, J. G.: Respiratory Care, A Guide to Clinical Practice. Philadelphia, J. B. Lippincott Co., 1977.

Demers, R. R.: IPPB treatments: Indications and alternatives. Respir. Care, *23*:758, 1978.

Morrison, D. R., Power, W. E., Boocks, R. D.: A proposal for the more rationale use of IPPB: volume orientation. Respir. Care, *21*:318, 1976.

Shapiro, B. A., Harrison, R. A., Trout, C. A.: Clinical Application of Respiratory Care. Chicago, Year Book Medical Publishers, Inc., 1975.

Wu, N., Miller, W. R., Code, R., and Richburg, P.: Intermittent positive pressure breathing in patients with chronic bronchopulmonary disease. Am. Rev. Pul. Dis., *71*:693, 1955.

CHAPTER FOUR

Chest Physiotherapy
Diane Blodgett, R.R.T.

GENERAL CONSIDERATIONS FOR
CHEST PHYSIOTHERAPY

This section deals with chest physiotherapy procedures, including postural drainage, chest percussion and vibration, rib springing, breathing exercises and coughing maneuvers. Not all chest physiotherapy procedures are covered here; those that are covered are those generally used in daily respiratory care.

The therapeutic objectives for chest physiotherapy procedures are the removal of secretions, reexpansion of lung tissue and breath control. Use of the procedures may be indicated for both the acute and the chronic respiratory patient. For those patients with retained secretions or collapse of lung tissue, postural drainage and/or chest percussion and vibration will aid in mobilization of secretions and opening of the airways. Coughing maneuvers also promote expectoration of sputum and the opening of airways. Breathing exercises benefit patients who are short of breath, need to minimize oxygen consumption, are anxious, or need to improve ventilation and muscle utilization.

Postural drainage relative contraindications include active tuberculosis, hemoptysis, untreated pneumothorax, head injury, recent history of cerebral vascular accident, fractured ribs or unstable chest wall and positional hypotension. Chest percussion, vibration and rib springing procedures are contraindicated in patients with empyema, rib fractures, hemoptysis, lung tumors, pain and fragile bony structures. There are no apparent contraindication to breathing exercises and there are really only precautions for coughing maneuvers. With the patient who has an incision, for example, care must be taken to guard against pain and stress on the incision site when coughing.

The criteria for termination of chest physiotherapy are a clear chest x-ray, normal ausculatory sounds, the ability to mobilize secretions, and/or the ability to normalize and control the breathing pattern.

POSTURAL DRAINAGE

Description

Postural drainage is the positioning of the patient to drain various lung segments.

Objective

To facilitate drainage and removal of secretions from the lung by taking advantage of gravitational forces.

Procedure

1. Approach the patient and explain the procedure.
2. Place the patient in proper position for drainage of specific lobe or segment (Tables 4-1, 4-2).
3. Leave the patient in this position for 15-20 minutes.
4. During this time period have the patient breathe deeply and cough.
5. Return the patient to the sitting position and ask him to cough.

Special Considerations

- Make sure the patient is comfortable.
- Support the patient's position with the use of pillows and bed rolls.
- Provide the patient with tissues and sputum cup for expectorated secretions.
- Have suction equipment available to remove secretions that may accumulate in the airway.
- The time of drainage may be reduced when percussion is used in conjunction with postural drainage.
- Do not attempt drainage immediately following a meal.
- Monitor vital signs carefully, especially in the head down position.

- Use breathing exercises and coughing maneuvers to facilitate loosening of secretions.
- Any adjunct therapy, such as aerosol, IPPB, or USN should be given before Chest PT.
- For patients who have generalized disease, start with the lower lobes, then clear the middle lobes, and finally the upper lobes. For small children, start with the upper lobes, then the middle lobes, and finally the lower lobes. For patients with localized disease, start with the involved segment, and then the segments that are disease free.

Hazards

- Positional hypotension.
- Increasing dyspnea.
- Overmobilization of secretions.
- Tipping may lead to further collapse in untreated pneumothorax.
- Increased intracranial pressure.

Maintenance

- Keep the patient comfortable during procedure.

(Text continues on p. 103.)

Table 4-1. General Positions For Chest Physical Therapy

Illustrations	Lung Lobes	Position	Instructions for Percussion & Vibration
Fig. 4-1	Upper lobes apical	Patient sitting in upright position.	Percuss and vibrate over uppermost portion of both sides of the chest to the nipple.
Fig. 4-2	Upper lobes posterior	Patient sitting with pillow in abdominal area and leaning forward.	Percuss and vibrate over posterior scapular area on both sides.
Fig. 4-3	Left lower lobe and lingula	Patient lying on right side with head down or pillow under hips.	Percuss and vibrate left side and back from axilla to bottom of ribs.
Fig. 4-4	Right middle & lower lobe	Patient lying on left side with head down or pillow under hips.	Percuss and vibrate right side and back from axilla to bottom of ribs.
Fig. 4-5	Lower lobes	Patient lying face down with pillow under lower chest and abdominal area.	Percuss and vibrate either side of vertebra from scapula to bottom of ribs.

Table 4-2. Positions For Drainage Of Specific Lung Segments

Illustrations	Lung Segment	Position	Instructions for Percussion & Vibration
Fig. 4-6	RUL Apical	Patient lying on back. Head raised to 30° angle.	Percuss and vibrate over uppermost portion of right back area.
Fig. 4-7	RUL Anterior	Patient lying flat on back, knees supported.	Percuss and vibrate over upper third of right side of chest.
Fig. 4-8	RUL Posterior	Patient sitting with pillow in abdominal area and leaning forward.	Percuss and vibrate over upper third of ribs on right side of back.

Fig. 4-6.

Fig. 4-7.

Fig. 4-8.

Fig. 4-3.

Fig. 4-4.

Fig. 4-5.

Fig. 4-1.

Fig. 4-2.

Table 4-2. Positions For Drainage Of Specific Lung Segments (Continued)

Illustration	Lung Segment	Position	Instructions for Percussion & Vibration
Fig. 4-9	RML Lateral medial	Patient lying on left side with head down, right side back ¼ turn, knees flexed.	Percuss and vibrate over right nipple area.
Fig. 4-10	RLL Superior	Patient lying on abdomen, hips supported.	Percuss and vibrate over middle third of ribs on right back.
Fig. 4-11	RLL Medial basal	Patient lying on abdomen with head down, hips supported, left side turned up slightly.	Difficult to percuss over appropriate area.
Fig. 4-12	RLL Anterior basal	Patient lying on back with head down, knees supported.	Percuss and vibrate over lower third of ribs on right side below the axilla.
Fig. 4-13	RLL Lateral basal	Patient lying on abdomen with head down, right side turned up slightly, hips supported.	Percuss and vibrate over middle third of ribs on right side.
Fig. 4-14	RLL Posterior basal	Patient lying on abdomen in head down position, hips supported.	Percuss and vibrate over lower third of ribs on right back.

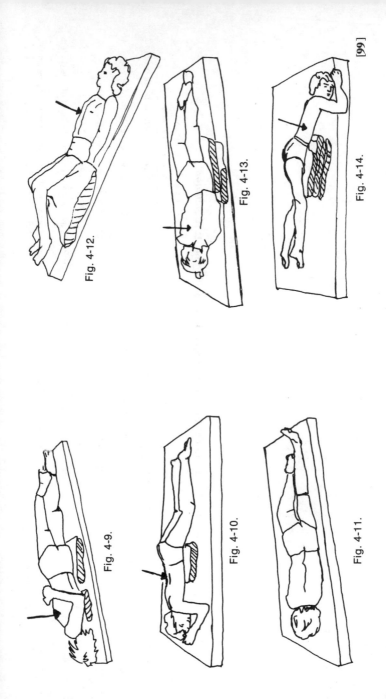

Fig. 4-12.

Fig. 4-13.

Fig. 4-14.

Fig. 4-9.

Fig. 4-10.

Fig. 4-11.

Table 4-2. Positions For Drainage Of Specific Lung Segments (Continued)

Illustrations	Lung Segment	Position	Instructions for Percussion & Vibration
Fig. 4-15	LUL Apical posterior	Patient lying on back, head raised to 30°.	Percuss and vibrate over uppermost portion of left back.
Fig. 4-16	LUL Anterior	Patient lying flat on back, knees supported.	Percuss and vibrate over upper third of left side of chest.
Fig. 4-17	LUL Lingula inferior-superior	Patient lying on right side with head down, left side back ¼ turn, knees flexed.	Percuss and vibrate over left nipple area.
Fig. 4-18	LLL Superior	Patient lying prone over pillow, hips supported.	Percuss and vibrate over middle third of ribs on left back.
Fig. 4-19	LLL Anterior basal	Patient lying on back with head down, knees supported.	Percuss and vibrate over lower third of ribs on left side below the axilla.

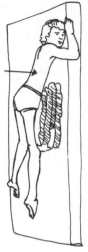

Fig. 4-18.

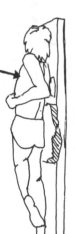

Fig. 4-17.

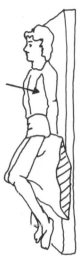

Fig. 4-19.

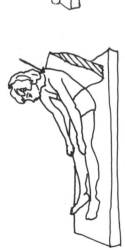

Fig. 4-15.

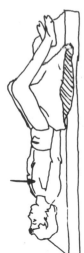

Fig. 4-16.

Table 4-2, Positions For Drainage Of Specific Lung Segments (Continued)

Illustrations	Lung Segment	Position	Instructions for Percussion & Vibration
Fig. 4-20	LLL Lateral basal	Patient lying on abdomen with left side turned up slightly, hips supported.	Percuss and vibrate over middle third of ribs on left side.
Fig. 4-21	LLL Posterior	Patient lying on abdomen in head down position, hips supported.	Percuss and vibrate over lower third of ribs on left side.

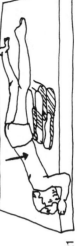

Fig. 4-21

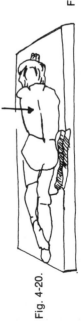

Fig. 4-20.

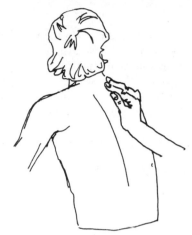

Fig. 4-22. Chest percussion—clapping (cupping).

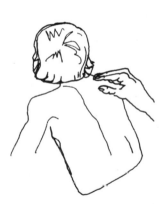

Fig. 4-23. Chest percussion—tapping.

CHEST PERCUSSION
(Clapping, cupping, tapping)

Description

Chest percussion is the use of the hands in the cupping, clapping, or tapping position over various segments of the chest wall.

Objective

To loosen and aid in the removal of lung secretions and to promote re-expansion of lung tissue.

Procedure

1. Approach the patient and explain the procedure.
2. Since this procedure is almost always used in conjunction with postural drainage, place the patient in the proper position for drainage of a specific lobe or segment (see Tables 4-1, 4-2).
4. Position hands for cupping, clapping or tapping over indicated area for each segment to be drained and percuss for 3-5 min.
5. After each position, have the patient breathe deeply and cough.
6. Return the patient to the sitting position and again ask him to cough.

Special Considerations

- Make sure the patient is comfortable.
- Use rhythmic percussion.
- Adjust amount of force to the individual patient but do not use forceful movements.
- Any adjuct therapy, such as aerosol, IPPB or USN should be given before chest PT.
- Do not percuss on bare skin.
- Do not percuss over kidneys, spine or female breasts.
- Any pain medication ordered should be given before chest PT to lessen discomfort.
- Do not percuss over area of tuberculosis, empyema, or cancerous tumors.
- Observe the same special considerations as for postural drainage.

Hazards

- Increased bronchospasm in asthmatics.
- Fractured ribs.
- May spread infection or tumor.
- May increase pulmonic bleeding or overmobilization of secretions.
- Note other hazards under postural drainage.

Maintenance

- Keep the patient comfortable during the procedure.

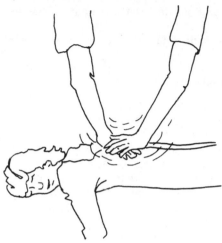

Fig. 4-24. Vibration.

CHEST VIBRATION

Description

Chest vibration is the placing of flat hands over area to be drained and vibrating the hands quickly during the expiratory phase of the respiratory cycle.

Objective

Aids in the loosening of secretions and the mobilization of secretions toward the trachea.

Procedure

1. Approach the patient and explain the procedure.
2. Since this procedure is almost always used in conjunction with postural drainage, place the patient in the proper position for drainage of a specific lobe or segment (see Tables 4-1, 4-2).
3. Place the flat of the hands over the area to be vibrated.
4. As the patient exhales, press firmly against the chest wall area; the contractions of the arm and shoulder muscle will create vibrations in the hands.
5. Vibrate for 3-5 minutes over each segment as indicated.

6. After each position, have the patient breathe deeply and cough.

7. Return patient to sitting position and again ask him to cough.

Special Considerations

- Make sure the patient is comfortable
- Do vibration only during expiration.
- Vibrate from the top of inspiration to end of expiration.
- Any adjunct therapy, such as aerosol, IPPB, or USN should be given before chest therapy.
- Do not vibrate over area of tuberculosis, empyema, or cancerous tumor.
- If pain medication is ordered, it should be given before chest therapy to lessen discomfort.
- Do not vibrate on bare skin.
- Observe special considerations for postural drainage.

Hazards

- Increased bronchospasm in asthmatics.
- May spread infection or tumor.
- Note other hazards under postural drainage.

Maintenance

- Keep the patient comfortable during the procedure.

RIB SPRINGING

Description

Rib springing is a maneuver that puts intermittent pressure on the chest wall during the expiratory phase.

Objective

Aids in loosening and transporting of secretions in the direction of the trachea.

Procedure

1. Approach the patient and explain the procedure.

2. Since the procedure is almost always used in conjunction with postural drainage, place the patient in the proper position for drainage of a specific lobe or segment.

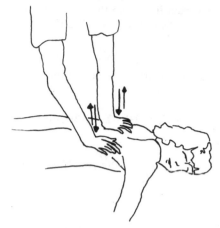

Fig. 4-25. Rib springing.

3. Place the flat of the hands over the area to be drained.

4. As the patient exhales, exert pressure and relax pressure 3-4 times with a spring-like action.

5. Repeat every other breath for one minute.

6. After each position, have the patient breathe deeply and cough.

7. Return patient to sitting position and again ask him to cough.

Special Considerations

- Use rib springing only during expiration.
- Any adjunct therapy such as aerosol, IPPB, or USN should be given before chest therapy.
- Do not use pressure over area of tuberculosis, empyema, or cancerous tumor.
- If pain medication is ordered, it should be given before chest therapy to lessen discomfort.
- Do not use rib springing on bare skin.
- Observe special considerations for postural drainage.

Hazards

- Increased bronchospasm in asthmatics.
- Do not use on patients with immobile chest wall (*i.e.*, patient with emphysema or increased A-P diameter).

- May increase pain in postop thoracic patient.
- Note other hazards under postural drainage.

Maintenance

- Keep the patient comfortable during the procedure.

BREATHING EXERCISES

Description

Breathing exercises utilize the patient's ability to control the volume and flow of air into the lungs.

Objectives

To normalize the pattern of breathing, improve ventilation, foster relaxation, and decrease oxygen consumption.

Procedure

Diaphragmatic
1. Approach the patient and explain the procedure.
2. Prepare the patient for this exercise by having him lie down and place one of his hands on his chest and one on his abdomen.
3. Instruct the patient to push his abdomen out against his hand as he inhales.
4. Direct the patient to pull his abdomen in as he exhales.

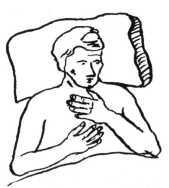

Fig. 4-26. Diaphragm breathing.

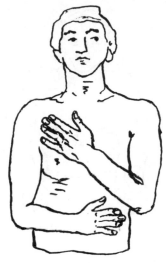

Fig. 4-27. Diaphragm breathing (standing).

5. Have him repeat this at a slightly slower than normal breathing rate.

6. When the patient has mastered this in the supine position, instruct him to follow this procedure in the sitting and standing positions.

Special Considerations

- Weights may be placed on the diaphragm to increase muscle strength.
- Use this procedure in combination with pursed-lip breathing.

Pursed-Lip

1. Approach the patient and explain the procedure.

2. Guide the patient through the breathing cycle.

3. Instruct the patient to take a normal inspiration through his nose.

4. Direct the patient to purse his lips and exhale.

5. Have the patient slow his exhalation, but do not allow him to prolong the expiratory phase extensively.

6. Repeat.

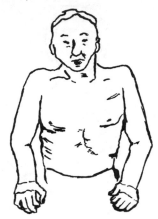

Fig. 4-28. Pursed-lip breathing.

Special Considerations

- Have the patient exhale against resistance by placing three fingers lightly over his mouth.
- Use this procedure in combination with diaphragmatic breathing.
- Have patient try to blow out candle while using pursed lip breathing.

Segmental (Costal)

1. Approach the patient and explain the procedure.
2. Place your hand over the affected area of the lung.
3. Instruct the patient to inhale.
4. Exert pressure on the affected area as the patient exhales.
5. Repeat.
6. Have the patient place his hand over the area and follow this procedure.

Special Considerations

- This technique is quite difficult for some patients to do.
- As the patient inhales, keep hand lightly on affected area.
- Patient must be cooperative and understand the instructions.
- All exercises should be taught in a quiet, calm atmosphere.
- Make sure the patient is comfortable.
- Use many positions (sitting, standing, reclining, walking) to teach the exercises.

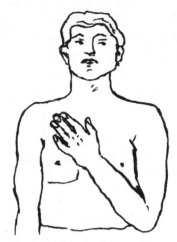

Fig. 4-29. Segmental breathing.

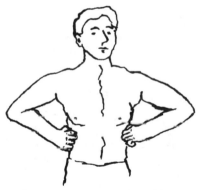

Fig. 4-30. Segmental breathing.

- Encouragement and reinforcement must be given to all patients while they are learning these techniques.

Hazards

- Overexertion when the patient forces the exercises.
- Increasing shortness of breath when patient attempts to do exercises rapidly.

Maintenance

• The therapist should coach the patient many times to insure that the exercises are being done correctly.

COUGHING MANEUVERS

Description

Coughing consists of a deep inhalation, closure of the glottis, contraction of respiratory muscles, the opening of the glottis and rapid expulsion of air.

Objective

Promotes expansion of lung tissue and mobilizes and clears the airway of secretions.

Procedure

1. Approach the patient and explain the procedure.
2. Position the patient for maximum effectiveness of maneuver, for most patients sitting is best, while for patients with respiratory muscle impairment head down is better.

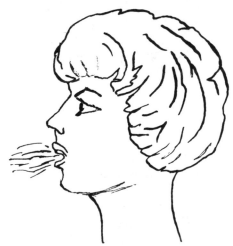

Fig. 4-31. Coughing.

3. Instruct the patient to take a deep breath in and hold it.
4. Then instruct the patient to contract the abdominal muscle and exhale rapidly while contracting his throat muscles.
5. Have the patient follow this pattern:
    Inhale—Hold—Contract muscles
    Exhale (sm. amt.)—Cough—Exhale (sm. amt.)
6. Repeat.

Special Considerations

• Splint patients with incision or pain.
• Pain medication should be given before respiratory therapy to decrease discomfort.
• For those patients who cannot take a deep breath, assisted ventilation should augment the attempt (IPPB, manual resuscitator).
• For those patients who cannot exhale forcibly, the therapist should place hands on the diaphragm and push during exhalation.
• Have the patient say "K,K,K" during the contracting of the throat muscles to assist the coughing effort.

Hazards

• Do not make the patient cough too long or hard.
• Venous return may be impaired.
• Precautions should be taken with those patients who have vascular abnormalities (CVA, aneurysms, etc.).
• Asthmatics should use caution when coughing.
• Uncontrollable coughing spasms may aggravate symptoms.

BIBLIOGRAPHY

Frownfeter, D.: Chest Physical Therapy and Pulmonary Rehabilitation. Chicago, Year Book Medical Publishers, Inc., 1978.
Gaskell, D. V., and Webber, B. A.: The Brompton Hospital Guide to Chest Physiotherapy. ed. 2. Oxford, Blackwell Scientific Publications, 1974.
Harris, J., and Bonita, J.: Indications and procedures for segmental bronchial drainage, Respir. Care, *20:*12, 1975.
Hillman, B. C.: The How and Why of Bronchial Drainage. Breon Laboratories, 1978.
Taylor, J. P.: Manual of Respiratory Therapy. St. Louis, C. V. Mosby Co., 1978.

CHAPTER FIVE

Airway Management
Diane Blodgett, R.R.T.

GENERAL CONSIDERATIONS FOR AIRWAY MANAGEMENT

The objectives of airway management are to provide and maintain a clear and patent airway and to protect the patient from aspiration. Airway management procedures include the insertion of artificial airways, the maintenance of those airways through suctioning, tracheal lavage and humidification, the use of cuff care techniques, trachcostomy care procedures and other techniques which insure that the objectives are met.

In this chapter, commonly used artificial airways are described and procedures for their insertion and use are provided. Charts giving characteristics of endotracheal and tracheostomy tubes are included. The anatomical airway and the care of tubes once they are in place are also topics included.

These techniques are common ones that all RT personnel should know and use. There are hazards involved with each technique just as there are benefits. These hazards are described under each individual procedure.

The criterion for termination of all these procedures is the return of the ability of the patient to maintain a clear and patent airway.

OROPHARYNGEAL AIRWAY

Description

Curved device made out of plastic, rubber, or metal that is inserted into the oral cavity. This rigid or semirigid airway conforms to the shape of the pharynx and is positioned externally by a flange.

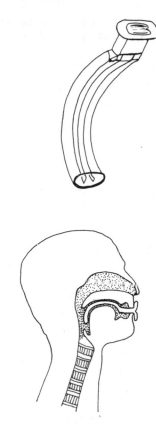

Fig. 5-1. Oropharyngeal airway.
(Modified from: Shapiro, B.:
Clinical Application of Respira-
tory Care. ed, 2. Chicago, Year
Book Medical Publishers, 1979.)

Objective

To maintain a patent airway and to facilate the removal of
secretions from the oropharynx.

Procedure

1. Hyperextend the neck.
2. Open the mouth either with a tongue depressor or a crossed
thumb and index finger.
3. Insert the tip of the airway into the mouth. (The curve of the
device should be at 180° to the mouth curve)
4. Gently rotate the airway upwards into position.
5. Position airway.

6. Clear oropharynx of secretions.
7. Tape airway into place.

Special Considerations

• Select the proper size.

> Sizes
> 00—Newborn
> 0—Infant
> 1—Child 1-3 years
> 2—Child 3-8 years
> 3—Large child-Small adult
> 4—Adult
> 5—Large Adult
> 6—Large Adult

• Tape the airway in place but do not occlude.
• Short term use only.
• Many types available—all have same objective.

Hazards

• Gagging and aspiration.
• Obstruction of airway if size of device is inappropriate.
• Gastric insufflation if airway is too large.
• Necrosis if airway is left in over extended time period.
• Occlusion of airway if mouth care not given.

Maintenance

• Keep oral pharyngeal cavity free from pooling secretions.
• Change airway if occluded with secretions.
• Reposition airway each hour.
• Provide mouth care hourly.

NASOPHARYNGEAL AIRWAY

Description

Hollow, slightly curved device of flexible rubber or plastic that is inserted into the nasal cavity. Usually cone-shaped to prevent total passage into the nasopharynx.

Objective

To maintain a patent airway.
To facilitate the removal of secretions from the nasopharynx.

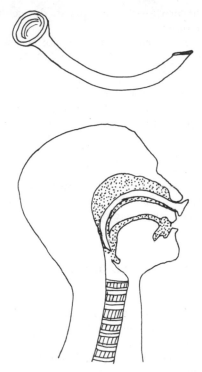

Fig. 5-2. Nasopharyngeal airway. (Modified from: Shapiro, B.: Clinical Application of Respiratory Care. ed. 2. Chicago, Year Book Medical Publishers, 1979.)

Procedure

1. Lubricate the tip of the airway with water-soluble jelly.
2. Gently pass the tip of the airway through the external nares, aiming downward.
3. Position the tube.
4. Check for adequate air exchange.
5. Secure the tube.

Special Considerations

- Select the proper size.
- If flange is not wide enough, insert large safety pin through the external end of the airway to prevent slippage.
- Short-term use only.

- Do not force the airway—if unable to pass device through one nostril, try the other.
- Useful for patients when oral cavity is not accessible.

Hazards

- Obstruction of airway from secretions.
- Gastric insufflation with airway that is too large.
- Necrosis of tissue if airway left in place over extended period of time.

Maintenance

- If possible reposition tube from one nostril to the other q8h.
- Keep airway free from secretions by providing adequate humidification and suctioning of secretions when necessary.
- Change airway if there is any question of obstruction.

ESOPHAGEAL OBTURATOR

Description

Emergency device that has an occluded, cuffed tube that is passed into the esophagus, holes in the upper portion of the tube for air passage, pilot balloon, a mask to cover the face and nose and a 15-mm. universal port to provide for support of ventilation by artificial means.

Objectives

To provide a patent airway, to prevent aspiration and to protect the airway.

Procedure

1. Place the patient in the supine position.
2. Clear the airway of foreign material.
3. Open the patient's mouth with a tongue blade and lift the jaw with thumb and index finger. Do not hyperextend the neck.
4. Following the curve of the oral cavity into the esophagus, slip the tube into the mouth and pass it into the stomach.
5. Inflate the pilot balloon with about 30 ml. air.
6. Attach manual resuscitator to 15-mm. adapter on mask or place mouth on adapter and begin ventilation.
7. Check placement of tube by listening over thoracic and abdominal area.

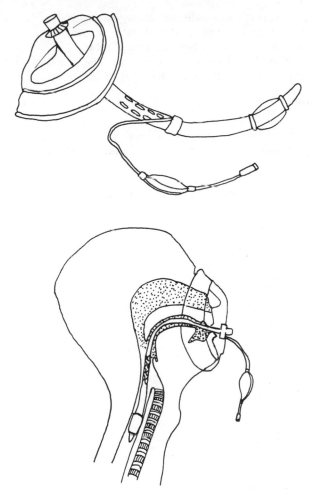

Fig. 5-3. Esophageal obturator. (Modified from: Shapiro, B.: Clinical Application of Respiratory Care. ed. 2. Chicago, Year Book Medical Publishers, 1979.)

Special Considerations

- Use only when endotracheal intubation is impossible.
- Do not use for severe face or head injuries.
- Breath sounds should be heard clearly when manual resuscitation provides a breath. No air should be heard entering the stomach.

- If patient starts to breath, mask may be removed.
- Have suction equipment at hand during extubation.
- Always deflate cuff before removal of tube.
- Do not use for children, conscious patients, or patients with damage to esophagus (*e.g.*, ingestion of caustic material).

Hazards

- Tracheal intubation.
- Trauma to the esophagus or airway.
- Gastric dilation if cuff is not inflated adequately.

Maintenance

- Clean and decontaminate after each use.

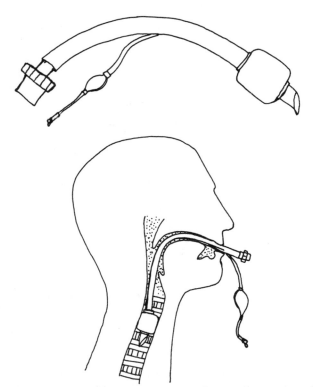

Fig. 5-4. Oral endotracheal tube. (Modified from: Shapiro, B.: Clinical Application of Respiratory Care. ed. 2. Chicago, Year Book Medical Publishers, 1979.)

ENDOTRACHEAL TUBES

Description

An endotracheal tube is a long, hollow, slightly curved airway inserted through the oral cavity into the trachea. This tube is usually made of rubber or semi-rigid plastic. The tubes may or may not be cuffed. There is a standard 15-mm. removal adapter for each size.

Objectives

To maintain a patent airway.

To relieve airway obstruction.

To prevent aspiration.

To provide an effective means of maintaining tracheobronchial hygiene.

To facilitate mechanical ventilation.

Procedure

Insertion (Orotracheal Intubation)

1. Place the patient in the supine position, with the neck hyperextended and the head slightly elevated above the shoulders.
2. Have the following equipment ready:
    a. suction equipment
    b. variety of different sized endotracheal tubes with adapters attached.
    c. Laryngoscope with straight or curved blades, sizes 1-4.
    d. Syringe to inflate cuff.
3. Select the appropriate tube size.
4. If tube has a cuff, test the cuff for proper inflation.
5. Select the blade and attach to the laryngoscope handle.
6. Insert the blade into the right side of the mouth, and move the tongue to the left.
7. Lift up slightly as the blade is moved forward.
8. Visualize the epiglottis and arytenoid cartilages.
9. Suction to clear secretions in the airway.
10. Insert the endotracheal tube along the right side of mouth.
11. Direct the tube, while still visualizing the cords through the opening of the glottis.
12. Advance the tube past the glottis so the top of the cuff is through the opening.

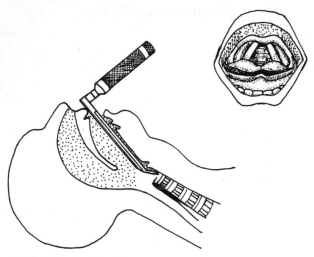

Fig. 5-5. Endotracheal intubation. (Modified from: Shapiro, B.: Clinical Application of Respiratory Care. ed. 2. Chicago, Year Book Medical Publishers, 1979.)

13. Remove the blade.

14. Inflate the cuff of the tube until a minimal or no-leak condition is met.

15. Inflate the lungs with a manual resuscitator to check for tube placement. (Bilateral, equal breath sounds should be heard).

Extubation

1. Approach the patient and explain the procedure.

2. Have equipment at hand to reintubate the patient if necessary.

3. Suction the airway to clear secretions.

4. Deflate the cuff and force the secretions upward by a manual breath.

5. Suction the upper airway to clear secretions.

6. Instruct the patient to take in a deep breath and cough.

7. As the patient coughs, pull the tube gently but smoothly from the patient's mouth.

8. Suction the mouth if necessary.

9. Watch the patient for signs of distress.

Special Considerations

- Lubricate the tube by applying water-soluble lubricant to the area of the cuff.
- Do not attempt to pass tube if the glottis is closed.
- Do not inflate cuff just by "feeling" the resistance against the syringe or the pressure in the pilot balloon.
- Monitor cuff pressure (see Chap. 7).
- Use sterile technique when suctioning patient.
- If bilateral equal breath sounds are not heard, the tube may
    a. Be in the esophagus, if no breath sounds are heard.
    b. Be in the right main stem bronchus, if sounds are only heard on right. If tube is in the right main stem bronchus, pull back on tube slightly and again listen for breath sounds.
- X-ray should be taken to check the placement of the tube.
- Mark a line on the endo tube so that if the tube does move it can easily be moved back to the correct position.
- Curved blade is placed into the vallecula, above the epiglottis.
- Straight blade is placed beyond the epiglottis to the left.
- Keep intubation equipment close by to reintubate the patient if accidental extubation occurs.

Hazards

- Misplacement of tube into esophagus or right main-stem bronchus.
- Traumatic intubation—chipping of teeth, bleeding, tissue damage to airway, rupture of trachea.
- Loss of communication route.
- Infection
- Hypoxia
- Bradycardia
- Obstruction of airway by placement of the distal tube orifice against the airway.
- Normal humidification mechanisms are bypassed.

Maintenance

- Keep airway patent by adequately humidifying the inspired air and suctioning secretions when necessary.
- Monitor cuff pressures.
- Change the placement of tube from one side of mouth to the other.
- Change bite block and tape and/or tie that hold tube in place.

General Characteristics of Endotracheal Tubes

1. Semi-rigid rubber or plastic tube.
2. Curved to conform to anatomical position.
3. Standard 15mm. universal adapter.
4. May be uncuffed or cuffed.
5. Radioopaque tip.
6. Length markers
7. Stylet may be used for insertion.
8. Beveled end.
9. Usually single patient use.

Table 5-1. Characteristics of Endotracheal Tubes: by Age

Adult	Pediatric
Cuff Type I—High residual volume— low-pressure cuff— (floppy)—less chance of pressure damage to trachea.	Uncuffed or cuffed Sizes 2.5-5.0mm May have tapered end (Cole). May have Tee configuration for use with circle ventilator set-up.
Type II—Low residual volume— high-pressure cuff— should only be used with minimal leak technique.	
Sizes 5.0-9.5mm.	

TRACHEOSTOMY TUBE

Description

A trach tube is a hollow, curved airway inserted into the tracheostomy site. It can be made of metal or synthetic material. It may or may not be cuffed. It usually has an obturator for ease of insertion.

Objective

To maintain an airway that bypasses an upper airway obstruction, to facilitate long-term mechanical ventilation, to provide an effective means of maintaining tracheobronchial hygiene, and (with a cuffed tube) to prevent aspiration.

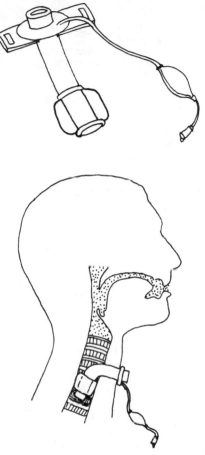

Fig. 5-6. Cuffed tracheostomy tube. (Modified from: Shapiro, B.: Clinical Application of Respiratory Care. ed. 2. Chicago, Year Book Medical Publishers, 1979.)

Procedure

Cleaning The Inner Cannula (for two-cannula tracheostomy tubes)

1. Approach the patient and explain the procedure.
2. Assemble the necessary equipment:
    a. Trach care tray—either disposable or hospital prepared.

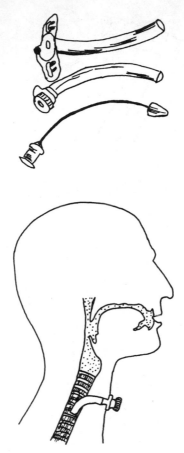

Fig. 5-7. Uncuffed tracheostomy tube. (Modified from: Shapiro, B.: Clinical Application of Respiratory Care. ed. 2. Chicago, Year Book Medical Publishers, 1979.)

     b. Solutions: 2-3% hydrogen peroxide, sterile distilled water, sterile normal saline.
     c. Suction equipment
     d. Scissors
     e. Sterile 4 × 4s
  3. Place patient in semi-Fowler's position.
  4. Wash hands with a germicidal soap.
  5. Prepare the tracheostomy care equipment.

a. Open sterile drape and position on work surface.

b. Open sterile 4 × 4s onto drape.

c. Fill two basins: one with sterile water, one with hydrogen peroxide.

6. Prepare suction equipment.

7. Preoxygenate the patient.

8. Suction inner cannula, if necessary.

9. Release lock of tracheostomy tube and remove inner cannula; place in basin of hydrogen peroxide.

10. Put on sterile gloves.

11. Clean inner cannula using cleaning brushes and pipe cleaners to remove mucus and crusts. Clean thoroughly.

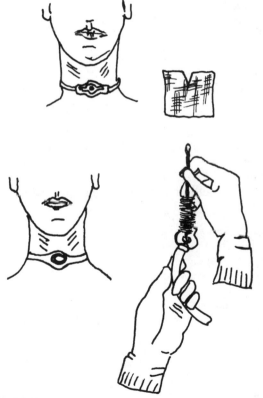

Fig. 5-8. Tracheostomy care-cleaning the inner cannula.

12. Place inner cannula in basin of water.

13. Clean flanges of outer cannula with moistened cotton swabs. Use sterile 4 × 4s to wipe away secretions that patient may expectorate.

14. Use sterile wipes to dry inner cannula.

15. Place cannula on drape.

16. Suction outer cannula, if necessary.

17. Gently reinsert inner cannula and lock in place.

18. Dispose of equipment.

Changing Tracheostomy Tube Bib

1. Remove and discard soiled bib.

2. Cleanse around the tracheostomy tube with 4 × 4s moistened with a sterile solution of water or normal saline.

3. Dry area.

4. Replace new bib gently to prevent dislodgement of tube.

5. Dispose of equipment.

Changing Tracheostomy Tube Ties

1. Prepare clean ties:
Fold one end of each tie over one inch and cut a slot $1/4 \times 1/3$ in. long.

2. Remove one soiled tie.

3. Insert uncut end through hole in side of flange of the outer cannula and thread this end through the slit on the other end; pull through until secure.

4. Repeat for second tie.

5. Secure a knot with the ties. For patient comfort, tie knot on side of neck.

Changing the Tracheostomy Tube

1. Approach the patient and explain the procedure. Oxygenate the patient.

2. Gather necessary equipment: suction equipment, gloves, 4 × 4s, new tube.

3. Suction the patient through the trach tube and then suction the oral-pharynx. Deflate cuff, have the patient cough (or inflate the lungs).

4. Again, oxygenate the patient.

5. The tube to be inserted should be prepared (*i.e.*, cuff checked, ties attached, obturator in place).

6. Put on sterile gloves.

7. Remove the trach bib and cut the trach ties carefully.

8. As the tube is being removed, have the patient exhale forcefully or cough.

9. Remove secretions from opening with sterile 4 × 4s.

10. Quickly, but gently, insert new tracheostomy tube into stoma, aiming back and downward.

11. Remove obturator and insert inner cannula, if necessary.

12. Secure tube in place.

13. Oxygenate the patient.

14. Suction the airway, if necessary.

Removing the Tracheostomy Tube

1. Approach the patient and explain the procedure.

2. Assemble the necessary equipment:
   a. Suction equipment.
   b. Sterile 4 × 4s.
   c. Tape.
   d. Gloves.

3. Place patient in semi-Fowler's position.

4. Wash hands.

5. Suction patient through the trach tube and then suction oropharynx. Deflate cuff.

6. Put on gloves and have 4 × 4s open and ready.

7. Cut the trach ties.

8. Have the patient cough as the trach is being removed.

9. Clear the stoma of any secretions with a 4 × 4.

10. Cover the stoma with a 4 × 4 and tape into place.

11. Check the patient's respirations and ability to clear the airway (have patient place fingers over gauze covering stoma and cough).

12. Dispose of equipment.

Special Considerations

- Change trach dressing when moist.
- Do not use dressing when drainage from fresh trach has diminished.
- Always keep a second trach tube at the bedside.
- Tape the obturator to the head of the bed.
- Do not use tracheostomy tubes with detachable cuffs, as they present a great hazard to the patient.
- Choose the trach tube that meets the needs of the patient (Tables 5-3, 5-4).

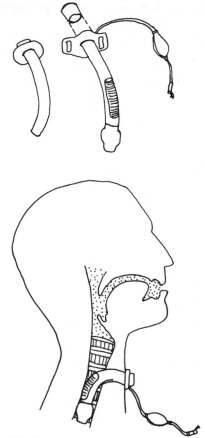

Fig. 5-9. Fenestrated tracheostomy tube.

- X-ray should be taken after the initial tracheostomy is done and the tube inserted. This will check the placement of the tube.
- Fenestrated tubes facilitate preparation for extubation.

Hazards

- Occlusion of airway.
- Herniation of the cuff.
- Tracheal erosion, stenosis, malacia.

- Infection.
- Displacement of tube.
- Subcutaneous emphysema.
- Hemorrhage
- Difficulty clearing secretions spontaneously.
- Loss of communication route.
- Natural humidification mechanisms are bypassed.

Maintenance

- Keep airway patent by adequately humidifying the inspired air and suctioning secretions when necessary.
- For tubes with an inner cannula, trach care should be given q2-q4 hours the first 24 hours, then q8h and p.r.n. thereafter.
- Change bib and ties when soiled.
- Change tube once a week or more often when indicated (*i.e.,* cuff blown).
- Monitor cuff pressures (see Chap. 7).

Table 5-2. Tube Size Conversion

French Size	Metric Size I.D.	Jackson Size
13	2.5	0
15	3.0	0
16.5	3.5	1
18	4.0	2
21	4.5-5.0	3
24	5.5	4
27	6.0-6.5	5
30	7.0	6
33	7.5-8.5	7
36	8.5	8
39	9.0-9.5	9
42	10.0	10

General Characteristics of Adult Trach Tubes

1. Curved or angled shape to facilitate insertion and removal.
2. Obturator with blunted end to facilitate insertion of outer cannula.
3. Cuffed tube used to prevent aspiration, to permit mechanical ventilation, to position cannula in center of trachea. Cuff—inflatable balloon on distal end of trach cannula—seals upper airway from lower airway.
4. Uncuffed tube used to maintain trachostomy over long period of time when there is no danger of aspiration or need for mechanical ventilation.

(*Text continues on p. 138.*)

Table 5-3. Specific Characteristics of Adult Trach Tubes

Specific Characteristics (Examples)

Name	Material	Cuff	Inner Cannula	Obturator	Sizes	Disposable	Special Considerations
Jackson trach tube	1. Silver 2. Stainless steel	No (can be attached, but not recommended)	Yes	Yes	3-10 mm. metal	No	Come in sets that do not have interchangeable parts. Lock keeps inner cannula in place. Trach care should be given PRN.
Air-lon trach tube	Nylon	No (can be attached, but not recommended)	Yes	Yes	3-8 mm. nylon	No	Come in sets that do not have interchangeable parts. Lock keeps inner cannula in place. Trach care should be given PRN.
Martin laryngectomy tube	1. Silver 2. Stainless steel 3. Nylon	No	Yes	Yes	8 mm. and 10 mm.	No	Come in sets that do not have interchangeable parts. Lock keeps inner cannula in place. Trach care should be given PRN. Tube larger and shorter than trach tube. Tube usually placed higher in neck.

| Lanz Controlled pressure cuff trach tube | Siliconized plastic (PVC) Coated in silicone | Yes—low pressure | Yes— disposable | Yes | 20 fr-40 fr (5-10 mm.) 7, 8, 9 mm. with disposable inner cannula | Yes | Fixed or adjustable neck-plate models. Coating on tube prevents crusting of secretions and blockage of airway. 15-mm. standard connection. Automatic pressure-regulating valve with external pressure control balloon. Radioopaque locating stripe on distal end of tube. |
| Portex blue line trach tube | Siliconized plastic (PVC) Impregnated with silicone | Yes—low pressure | No | Yes | 24 fr-39 fr (6-10 mm.) | Yes | Impregnated—no crusting on inside and outside of tube. 15-mm. standard connection. One way valve to inflate pilot balloon. Double cuffed tube available. Radioopaque blue line makes tube easy to identify on x-ray. |

(Continued on overleaf)

[133]

Table 5-3. Specific Characteristics of Adult Trach Tubes (continued)
Specific Characteristics (Examples)

Name	Material	Cuff	Inner Cannula	Obturator	Sizes	Disposable	Special Considerations
Kamen-Wilkinson trach tube Fome-Cuf Tube	Silicone & Poly-urethane	Yes—low pressure	No	Yes	#5–#9	Yes	Coating on tube prevents crusting of secretions and blocking of airway. 15-mm. standard connection. Radio-opaque tip for ease of location on X-ray. To insert tube, air is first withdrawn from cuff; tube is then inserted and cuff is allowed to inflate when port is opened to atmosphere. Do not use trach talk with this type of tube. The airway will be completely occluded!

National catheter	Plastic (PVC) Impregnated with silicone	Yes—low pressure	No	Yes	5-10 mm.	Yes	Single safety strap prevents disconnection. Radioopaque tip to tip 15-mm. standardized connector with swivel adapter and suction port, one-way inflation valve.
Shiley PRV-LPC	PVC	Yes—low pressure	Yes	Yes	4, 6, 8, 10 (5-9 mm.) 26-39 fr	Yes	During cuff inflation, any pressure above 25mm. Hg in cuffs is vented to atmosphere. Once relief valve is closed, cuff pressure can increase as patient or tube changes position. Trach care should be given PRN. Radio-opaque.
Dow Corning Silastic	Silicone rubber	Some with & some without cuffs	Yes	Some with Some without	0-9	Yes	Radioopaque, flexible. Trach care should be given PRN for those tubes with inner cannula.

Table 5-4. Specific Characteristics of Pediatric Trach Tubes

Name	Material	Cuff	Inner Cannula	Obturator	Sizes	Disposable	Special Considerations
Portex infants trach tube	Transparent PVC	No	No	No	3.1-6.0 mm.	Yes	Is *not* radioopaque. Small lumen—keep clear of secretions. Shape of flange and tube designed and adapted to anatomy of newborn or small infant.
Shiley Pediatric trach tube	PVC	No	No	Yes	00-3 (3.1-4.8 mm.)	Yes	15-mm. standard connector. Radioopaque. Ninety degree distal end, cut to minimize the possibility of blocking against anterior wall. Anatomically shaped flange and cannula for pediatric use. Small lumen—keep clear of secretions.
Rusch flexible trach tube	PVC with stainless steel spiral	No	No	Intubating tube	3-6 mm.	Yes	Standard 15-mm. connector. Fully

						Comments
						flexible tube that adapts to any change in position of trachea. Adjustable flange with lock ring that prevents movement when tube in place. Spiral—radioopaque. Small lumen size—keep clear of secretion. Intubating guide is also suction catheter.
Jackson trach tube	1. Silver 2. Stainless steel	No	Yes	Yes	00-3 (3.1-4.8 mm.)	No	Comes in sets that do not have interchangeable parts. Lock keeps inner cannula in place. Small lumen—keep clear of secretions. Trach care should be given p.r.n.

Characteristics of Pediatric Trach Tubes

1. Shape designed especially for the size of the patient.
2. Usually no inner cannula because of the tube size.
3. No cuff.
4. Obturator may or may not be available for insertion.
5. Correct size must be chosen. Too large—pressure necrosis, too small—large leak.

TRACHEOSTOMY BUTTON

Description

A short, straight, hollow plastic tube inserted into the tracheostomy stoma. This device does not occlude the airway and allows unobstructed airflow between the upper and lower airways.

Objective

To maintain a tracheostomy stoma.

Procedure

Determining the Size
1. Select a trach button the same size (external diameter) as the patient's tracheostomy.
2. Measure length of stoma. Insert a marked curette into the stoma and measure from the anterior wall of the trachea to the skin surface.
3. Place spacers on trach button to adjust length of cannula.

Insertion of Trach Button
1. Approach the patient and explain the procedure.
2. Lubricate the button with a water-soluble jelly.
3. Gently insert the button into the stoma.
4. Insert closure plug into button.
5. Check for proper placement and fit. Should be firm and secure.

Removal of Trach Button
1. Approach the patient and explain the procedure.
2. Remove the closure plug.
3. Gently pull the cannula straight out.

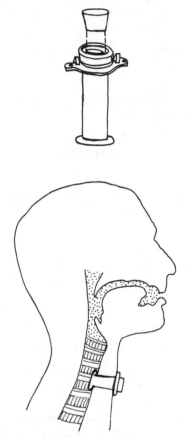

Fig. 5-10. Tracheostomy button. (Modified from: Shapiro, B.. Clinical Application of Respiratory Care. ed. 2. Chicago, Year Book Medical Publishers, 1979.)

Special Considerations

- Keep stoma site clean and dry.
- Make sure appropriate size button is inserted.
- Adapter available with 15-mm. fitting to use with various RT treatment modalities.
- Make sure button is sterile before using.
- Sizes 27-42 French.

Hazards

- Infection.
- Localized irritation.

Maintenance

- Remove and clean button twice a week with hydrogen peroxide and sterile water.

TRACH TALK

Description

Device attached to tracheostomy tube which allows the patient to talk.

Objective

To allow a patient with a tracheostomy tube in place to speak without placing his finger over the tube opening.

Procedure

1. Approach the patient and explain the procedure and device.
2. Deflate the cuff for patients with a cuffed tracheostomy tube.
3. Check the patency of the upper airway by having the patient occlude the opening to the trach.
4. Ask the patient to speak.
5. If the patient can speak, attach the trach talk to the tube via the standard 15-mm. adapter, or fit the tube with an adapter.
6. For continuous aerosol therapy, large-bore tubing can be attached to either inlet.

Special Considerations

- Patient can be suctioned through port or by removal of trach talk.
- Aerosol therapy can be administered concurrently with the use of this device.
- Do not use this device with tight-fitting trach tube, trach tube with cuff inflated or with a patient who has an airway obstruction above the tracheostomy tube.
- Fits most standard trach tube fittings.
- Check the patient frequently during initial trial for signs of increased work of breathing or obstruction.

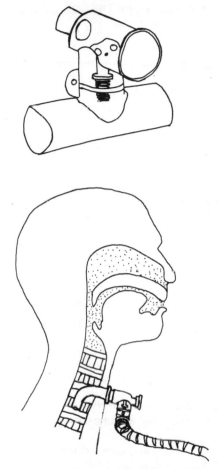

Fig. 5-11. Trach talk. (Modified from: Shapiro, B.: Clinical Application of Respiratory Care. ed. 2. Chicago, Year Book Medical Publishers, 1979.)

Hazards

- Occlusion of airway.
- Increased work of breathing.

Maintenance

- Disposable device that can be disassembled for decontamination.

NASAL OR ORAL PHARYNGEAL SUCTIONING

Description

Nasal pharyngeal suctioning is the removal of secretions from the lower and upper airway by exerting a vacuum through a suction catheter that is placed proximal to the secretions. This catheter is positioned directly via the nasal or oral cavity into the pharynx or trachea.

Objectives

To maintain a patent airway.

To remove secretions from those patients who are unable to expectorate.

Procedure

1. Approach the patient and explain the procedure.
2. Obtain necessary equipment (suction source, regulator bottle, connecting tubing, sterile suction catheter, sterile gloves, sterile saline or water, sterile basin, water-soluble jelly).
3. Wash hands.
4. Preoxygenate the patient by increasing the FIO_2 and position the patient (usually in semi-Fowler's).
5. Using aseptic technique, fill basin with sterile water or saline.
6. Open catheter and glove(s).
7. Turn on regulator and adjust suction source to appropriate vacuum.
8. Put on glove(s) and attach catheter to connecting tubing.
9. Lubricate catheter with jelly.
10. Insert catheter through the nares along the base of the nasal cavity (or through oral cavity).
11. Having the patient breathe slowly with his mouth open.
12. As the patient inhales, advance the catheter twisting it slightly.
13. When the patient coughs as you advance the catheter, the trachea has been reached.
14. Place thumb over the control port of the catheter and apply suction.
15. Release thumb and withdraw catheter slightly.

16. Again apply suction and release.

17. Withdraw catheter, suction, release suction in this order until catheter is removed.

18. Clear catheter and tubing with sterile solution.

19. Reoxygenate the patient and suction again if necessary.

Special Considerations

- Disposable suction kits may contain any or all of these sterile items: gloves, catheter, water, basin.
- Do not suction for more than 15-20 seconds.
- Always preoxygenate or hyperinflate the patient before suctioning.
- Use the appropriate size of catheter (see Table 5-5).
- Suction catheters should never be reused.
- Coude catheter may facilitate the removal of secretions from the right main stem bronchus.
- Turn patient's head to left to suction right bronchus.
- Turn patient's head to right to suction left bronchus.

Average Range of Vacuum Settings for Various Age Groups

Infants:
   3-5 in Hg (portable suction)
   60-100 mm. Hg (wall)

Children:
   5-10 in Hg (portable)
   100-120 mm. Hg (wall)

Adults:
   7-15 in Hg (portable)
   120-150mm. Hg (wall)

Hazards

- Hypoxia.
- Cardiac arrythmias.
- Bradycardia.
- Airway mucosal trauma.
- Infection.
- Atelectasis.

Maintenance

- Dispose of equipment after each use.

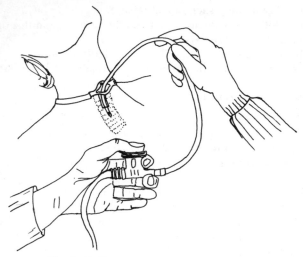

Fig. 5-12. Tracheobronchial suctioning.

TRACHEOBRONCHIAL SUCTIONING

Description

Tracheobronchial suctioning is the removal of secretions from the lower airway by exerting a vacuum through a catheter that is placed proximal to the secretions. This procedure is accomplished directly through an endotracheal, tracheostomy or laryngectomy tube.

Objective

To maintain a patent airway.

To remove secretions from those patients with artificial airways who are unable to clear their own airways.

Procedure

1. Approach the patient and explain the procedure.
2. Obtain necessary equipment (suction source, regulator bottle, connecting tubing, sterile suction, catheter, sterile gloves, sterile saline or water, sterile basin).
3. Wash hands.

4. Preoxygenate the patient by increasing the F_{IO_2} or sighing the patient.

5. Position patient (usually semi-Fowler's).

6. Using aseptic technique, fill basin with sterile saline or water.

7. Turn on regulator and adjust suction source to appropriate vacuum setting.

8. Put on glove(s) and attach catheter to connecting tubing.

9. Remove O_2 administrating device.

10. Pass catheter through opening of endotracheal or tracheostomy tube without applying suction.

11. When level to be suctioned is reached, place thumb over the control port of the catheter and apply suction.

12. Release thumb and withdraw catheter slightly.

13. Again apply suction and release.

14. Withdraw catheter, suction, release suction in this order until catheter is removed.

15. Clear catheter and tubing with sterile solution.

16. Reoxygenate patient and suction again if necessary.

Special Considerations

- Disposable suction kits may contain any or all of these sterile items: gloves, catheters, water basin.
- Do not suction for more than 15-20 seconds.
- Always preoxygenate or hyperinflate the patient before suctioning.
- Use appropriate size catheter (Table 5-5).
- Suction catheters should never be reused.
- Coude catheter may facilitate the removal of secretions from the right main stem bronchus.
- To loosen secretions, 3-5 ml. of sterile saline can be instilled into the endotracheal, tracheostomy or laryngectomy tubes before suctioning.
- The patient who is being artificially ventilated can be reconnected to the ventilator and given 2-3 hyperinflation breaths following the instillation and preceding the suction procedure.
- For the patient who is not being ventilated, 2-3 hyperinflation breaths by manual resuscitator with oxygen, following the instillation and preceding the suction procedure, is recommended.

Table 5-5. Suction Catheter Sizes for Age Groups and Artificial Airways

Oral-Nasal Suctioning		Trachealbronchial Suction (tube in place)	
Age	Catheter Size	Tube Size I.D.	Catheter Size
Infants	5 fr	2.5–4.0	5
Children	6-12 fr	4.5–5.0	6
Adults	12-16 fr	5.5–6.5	8–10
		7.0–8.0	12
		8.0–9.5	14
		10.0	16–18

- Turn patient's head to left to suction right bronchus.
- Turn patient's head to right to suction left bronchus.

Hazards

- Hypoxia.
- Cardiac Arrythmia.
- Atelectasis.
- Bradycardia.
- Infection.
- Airway mucosal trauma.

Maintenance

- Dispose of equipment after each use.

MINIMAL-LEAK TECHNIQUE

Description

This technique allows a small amount of air to escape from the lower airway to the upper airway around the inflated cuff of an endotracheal or tracheostomy tube.

Objective

To inflate the cuff of an endotracheal or tracheostomy tube to the point where a small amount of air is allowed to escape around it. This technique minimizes the chances of tracheal wall damage from an overinflated cuff.

Procedure

1. Approach the patient and explain the procedure.
2. Place a stethoscope diaphragm on the patient's trachea.

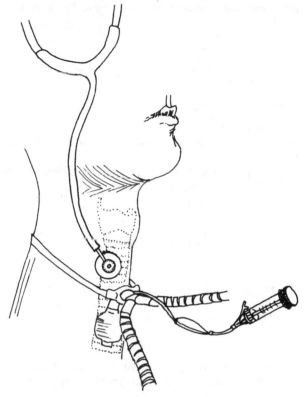

Fig 5-13. Minimal-leak technique.

3. Start to inject air into the inflating tube, which is connected to the endotracheal of tracheostomy tube cuff.

4. Cycle the ventilator and inject air into the inflating tube.

5. At the end of inspiration, listen over the trachea for a small air leak.

6. If no leak is heard, repeat the procedure, while slightly deflating the cuff.

7. Check pressure in cuff (see Chap. 7).

Special Considerations

• Can only be used on patients using PEEP or C-PAP, when ventilators are adjusted to compensate for the leak.

- Adjust ventilator settings to compensate for leak for all patients.

Hazards

- Aspiration around cuff.
- Hypoventilation.

Maintenance

- Check leak routinely.
- If there is no apparent air flow around cuff or air leak is large, repeat procedure.
- Check cuff volume and pressure q2h, when patient is repositioned and when reinflating cuff.
- Do not exceed pressures of 25 mm. Hg.

NO-LEAK TECHNIQUE

Description

This technique totally blocks the passage of air between the upper and lower airway. No air is allowed to pass around the endotracheal or tracheostomy tube when the cuff is inflated.

Objective

To totally occlude the space between the tracheal wall and the cuff on a cuffed endotracheal or tracheostomy tube.

Procedure

1. Approach the patient and explain the procedure.
2. Place a stethoscope diaphragm on the patient's trachea.
3. Start to inject air into the inflating tube which is connected to the endotracheal or tracheostomy tube cuff.
4. Cycle the ventilator and inject air into the inflating tube.
5. At the end of inspiration, listen over the trachea for a small leak. No air movement should be heard.
6. Repeat procedure until air leak is eliminated.
7. Check pressure in cuff (see Chap. 7).

Special Considerations

- Technique should only be used where cuff pressures and volumes are carefully monitored.

- May be indicated for 1) patients on PEEP or C-PAP, 2) patients who aspirate, and 3) patients with decreased lung compliance.

Hazards

- Erosion of the tracheal wall due to high cuff pressures.

Maintenance

- Check cuff volume and pressure q2h, when patient is repositioned and when reinflating cuff.
- Do not exceed pressures of 25 mm. Hg.

SPUTUM INDUCTION

Description

The patient is given a heated aerosol or ultrasonic nebulization treatment to induce a productive cough. A sterile specimen is collected.

Objectives

To assist the patient in raising sputum; to obtain a specimen of sputum for examination.

Procedure

1. Approach the patient and explain the procedure.
2. Administer aerosol therapy with hypertonic saline for 20-30 minutes.
3. After 10 minutes, encourage the patient to cough.
4. If the patient can raise any sputum, it should be expectorated into a sterile specimen container.
5. Continue aerosol therapy up to 30 minutes to induce a productive cough.
6. Label specimen and send to laboratory immediately.

Special Considerations

- Respiratory therapy personnel should wear mask and gown when collecting specimen from contagious patient.
- Collect specimen in a sterile cup.
- Do not use bacteriostatic agent in aerosolized solution.
- Label specimen with name, date, time and source of specimen.

Hazards

• Possible spreading of contagious desease.

Maintenance

• Send specimen to laboratory immediately.
• See aerosol therapy treatment procedure.

SPECIMEN TRAP

Description

This device allows the trapping of secretions in a sterile specimen container during a suctioning procedure.

Objective

To collect, by suctioning, a sterile specimen for examination.

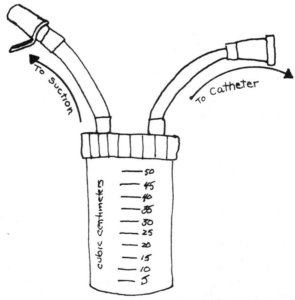

Fig. 5-14. Specimen trap.

Procedure

1. Assemble suction equipment.
2. Place trap in line with suction catheter and suction tubing (Fig. 5-14).
3. Turn on and adjust suction control.
4. Suction the patient using an aseptic technique.
5. Collect specimen in the vial.
6. After sample is obtained, remove suction catheter and tubing from trap.
7. Seal trap by connecting the two open parts together.
8. Label trap and send specimen to laboratory immediately.

Special Considerations

- Some traps may have suction catheter attached, necessitating the replacement of catheter cap with a plain cap.
- If secretions are thick, rinse catheter clear with a small amount of saline.
- Label specimen with name, date, time and source of specimen.

Hazards

- Spread of infection.

Maintenance

- Dispose of all materials after use.
- Send specimen to laboratory immediately.

BIBLIOGRAPHY

Burton, G. G., Gee, G. N., and Hodgkin, J. G. (eds.): Respiratory Care, A Guide to Clinical Practice. Philadelphia, J. B. Lippincott, 1977.

Long, J.: Tracheostomy Care Handbook. Wilmington, Mass., Portex Division of Smith Industries, Inc., 1976.

Slonin, N. B., and Schneider, N.: Pediatric Respiratory Therapy. New York, Glenn Educational Medical Services, Inc., 1974.

Wood, L. (ed.): Nursing Skills for Allied Health Services. Philadelphia, W. B. Saunders, 1977.

Young, J. and Crocker, D. (eds.): Principles and Practice of Respiratory Therapy. ed. 2. Chicago, Yearbook Publishers, 1976.

TECHNICAL INFORMATION

Portex Division, Smith Industries, Inc., Wilmington, Mass.
Rusch, Inc., New York, New York 10010
Shiley Laboratories, Inc., Santa Ana, Calif. 92711
Extra Corporeal Medical Specialists, Inc., King of Prussia, Pa. 19406
Ditmar and Penn Corp., Philadelphia, Pa. 19144
Biovena Surgical Instrument, McGaw Laboratories, Division of Hospi-
    tal Supply Corp., Irvine, Calif.
National Catheter Corp., Argyle, New York 12809
Dow Corning, Medical Products Division, Midlance, Michigan

CHAPTER SIX

Assisted Ventilation: An Integrated Approach

Frank Smith, B.S. R.R.T.
Carl Wiezalis, M.S. R.R.T.

GENERAL CONSIDERATIONS FOR ASSISTED VENTILATION

The recent polularity of ventilator care places a significant responsibility on the respiratory care clinician. The role performed by these individuals is a critical part of the overall evaluation and management of acutely and chronically ill patients who need mechanical ventilatory assistance. The respiratory clinician must have a thorough understanding of indications, complications, and weaning criteria for assisted ventilation, as well as an in depth understanding of the mechanical function of the ventilator selected to assist the patient. Shapiro, *et al.* state that the clinical goals of ventilator care are

1. to provide the pulmonary system with the mechanical power to maintain physiologic ventilation.
2. to manipulate the ventilatory pattern and airway pressures for purposes of improving the efficiency of ventilation and/or oxygenation.
3. to decrease myocardial work by diminishing the work of breathing and improving ventilatory efficiency.

These goals state clearly the overall physiologic benefits which can be achieved through mechanically assisted ventilation. The respiratory clinician must keep in mind at all times that assisted ventilation is a supportive therapeutic modality and not a cure-all for the primary pathology leading to the need for mechanically assisted ventilation. It is to be hoped, however, that if properly employed and managed, it will provide the time to reverse the primary pathology.

The physiologic benefits of ventilator care become the basis for the guidelines indicating the need for mechanically assisted

Table 6-1. Guidelines for Ventilatory Support in Adults

Datum	Normal Range	Tracheal Intubation and Ventilation Indicated
Mechanics:		
Respiratory Rate	12-20	>35
Vital capacity (ml./kg. of body weight)	65-75	<15
FEV_1 (ml./kg. of body weight)	50-60	<10
Inspiratory force (cm. H_2O)	75-100	<25
Oxygenation:		
Pa_{O_2} (mm. Hg)	75-100 (air)	<70 (on mask O_2)
$P_{(A-aD)O_2}$ 1.0 (mm. Hg)	25-65	>450
Ventilation		
Pa_{CO_2} (mm. Hg)	35-45	>55
$\dot{V}_D/\dot{V}_T$	0.25-0.40	>0.60

(Pontoppidan, H., et al.; Acute Respiratory Failure in the Adult. Boston, Little, Brown and Co., 1973, p. 60.)

ventilation (MAV). Pontoppidan, *et al.* emphasized the application of physiologic concepts and data to the clinical setting when determining the need for MAV and the management of patients receiving MAV. Table 6-1 states the guidelines for ventilatory support for adults as described by Pontoppidan, *et al.*

These guidelines exclude some of the physiologic data for chronic CO_2 retainers. With these individuals it is important to evaluate pH and Pa_{O_2} levels in the arterial blood rather than $\dot{V}_D/\dot{V}_T$ and Pa_{CO_2} levels (which are normally elevated in CO_2 retainers). Chronic CO_2 retainers will demonstrate their inability to provide ventilation for themselves during acute exacerbations, through hypoxemia and acidosis ($pH < 7.35$).

After collecting the physiologic data and determining if it falls within the guidelines indicating mechanically assisted ventilation, the respiratory clinician must draw from a completely new body of knowledge which allows for the selection of a mechanical ventilator. The integration of the physiologic concepts stressed by Pontoppidan, *et al.* becomes extremely obvious when the physiologic homeostasis of the patient is dependent upon a mechanical ventilator. The respiratory clinician must possess the same thorough understanding of the ventilator chosen to support a patient as he has of the guidelines used to indicate the need for MAV.

Confusion exists in literature available today describing the various classifications or descriptions of ventilators. Several classification techniques have been published and no one is better than the other. It becomes extremely important, however, that the respiratory clinician does not overlap or share classification systems. The respiratory clinician must concentrate on one system and become completely familiar with that system so as to apply it in the clinical setting. This author will present one common classification system which will help a clinician to select and operate any ventilator available on the market today, provided the classification is available.

Every ventilator has four basic phases it must complete in providing a ventilatory cycle to a patient. These four phases include:

1. Inspiratory phase
2. Inspiratory → Expiratory phase
3. Expiratory phase
4. Expiratory → Inspiratory phase

Table 6-2. Phases of a Ventilator

Phase I	Phase II	Phase III	Phase IV
Inspiratory phase Generating force	Inspiratory → Expiratory phase Cycling mechanism	Expiratory phase Retard, PEEP, NEEP, ZEEP	Expiratory → Inspiratory phase Mode of ventilation

Positive pressure ventilators are divided into 3 types:

1. Constant flow generators
2. Nonconstant flow generators
3. Pressure generators

Constant flow generators utilize a high generating pressure to maintain a constant flow of gas between the ventilator and the patient's airways. Figure 6-1 demonstrates the flow pattern presented by constant flow generators. Figure 6-2 represents the pressure in the lungs during the inspiratory phase with constant flow generators.

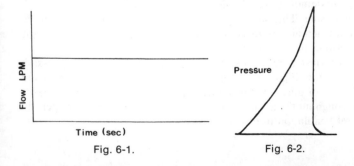

Fig. 6-1.   Fig. 6-2.

Constant flow generators lend themselves nicely to treatment for patients with pure compliance problems. The high generating force maintained during the inspiratory phase overcomes ↓ compliance, thus allowing lung inflation. In most pulmonary cases, however, airway resistance is increased and compliance is decreased. The constant flow rate during the inspiratory phase is a direct result of the high generating force and will result in less peripheral ventilation in areas of the lung where airway resistance is increased. This concept will be further explained later in this chapter.

Figure 6-3 represents the flow pattern during the inspiratory phase of a non-constant flow generator. The sine wave pattern is very similar to the normal inspiratory flow pattern.

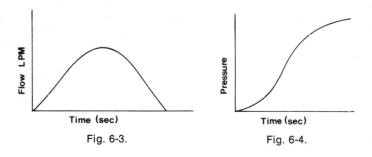

Fig. 6-3.   Fig. 6-4.

Figure 6-4 represents the proximal airway pressure during the inspiratory phase with nonconstant flow generators. The flow pattern will not change from breath to breath even when lung characteristics change. Thus, when airway resistance ↑ and compliance ↓, the actual volume delivered to the patient could be decreased. The second half of the nonconstant flow generator curve demonstrates the flow rate decreasing as lung pressure is increasing. This situation will result in more peripheral ventilation when airway resistance is elevated than is provided by the constant flow generator.

The last type of positive pressure generator is the pressure generator. Figure 6-5 represents the flow pattern of a pressure generator during the inspiratory phase. The flow rate decreases throughout the inspiratory phase, which results in better peripheral ventilation in obstructed airways.

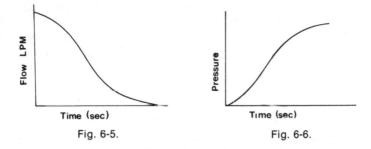

Fig. 6-5.　　　　　　　　　　　　Fig. 6-6.

As the flow rate decreases and lung pressure increases, turbulent flow at the site of obstruction is minimized, and thus more volume is delivered beyond the obstruction (Fig. 6-6). Poiseuille's Law demonstrates this phenomenon.

Part *(2)* in Figure 6-7 demonstrates all the constants removed from Poiseuille's Law and r^4 (radius of airway) ↓ , thus increasing airway resistance when $\dot{V}$ remains constant as with constant flow generators. The P (back pressure) is increased, resulting in less volume passing by the obstructed area. Part *(3)* represents the pressure generator phenomenon; where r^4 decreases, $\dot{V}$ also decreases, thus diminishing the degree of back pressure and resulting in better ventilation past the obstruction. The popularity of pressure generators is based on this phenomenon.

(1)
$$P = \frac{n8L\,\dot{V}}{\pi\,r^4}$$

(2) $\uparrow P \cong \dfrac{\dot{V}}{r^4 \downarrow}$　　constant

(3) $P \cong \dfrac{\dot{V}\downarrow}{r^4 \downarrow}$

P = Pressure
n = Viscosity
L = Length
$\dot{V}$ = Flow (ml./sec.)
π = Constant
r^4 = Tube radius

Fig. 6-7. Poiseuille's Law.

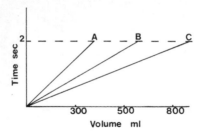

Fig. 6-8. Delivery volume changes that can occur in the lung when using time-cycled machines. (*A*) ↓ compliance or ↑ airway resistance. (*B*) Normal compliance and airway resistance. (*C*) ↑ compliance or ↓ airway resistance.

Phase II of the ventilator cycle ends inspiration and begins expiration. Three things can result in inspiration ending, thus allowing exhalation to begin: time, volume and pressure. These three factors are considered the cycling mechanisms of ventilators.

A time-cycled ventilator is one in which, after a preset period of time, inspiration ends. The volume and pressure are variable and can only be considered limiting factors. For example, if a time-cycle machine has a pressure relief valve set at 50 cm.H_2O the inspiratory phase will last the length of time established. If ;50 cm.H_2O is reached, however, the volume will be eliminated outside the patient's ventilator system and the pressure limited to 50 cm.H_2O. Figure 6-8 demonstrates the volume delivery changes that can occur with changes in lung characteristics when using time-cycled machines.

It is obvious that a person with normal lung characteristics and one with ↑ lung compliance or ↓ airway resistance will receive more volume than a person with ↓ compliance or ↑ airway resistance. Most pulmonary complications resulting in the need for mechanically assisted ventilation fall into category *A*. Therefore, the volume delivered to the patient must be continuously monitored with time-cycled machines in order to assure adequate alveolar ventilation.

Volume-cycled ventilators end inspiration after a preset volume has been delivered to the patient. Pressure and time are the limiting factors which must be considered with volume-cycled machines. Assuming time and pressure limits are not exceeded, the volume selected will be delivered each breath to

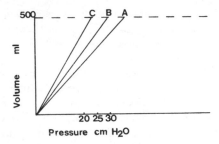

Fig. 6-9. Changes in pressure that occur in lung when using volume-cycled machines. *(A)* ↓ compliance or ↑ airway resistance. *(B)* Normal compliance and airway resistance. *(C)* ↑ compliance or ↓ airway resistance.

the patient. This allows for a more accurate regulation of alveolar ventilation. Figure 6-9 demonstrates the changes in pressure that occur with lung characteristic changes when using volume-cycled machines.

The third type of cycling mechanism for ventilators is pressure. Pressure-cycled ventilators end inspiration when a preset pressure has been reached during the inspiratory phase. Volume and time become the variables which must be considered. Changes in lung characteristics will alter the volume delivered from breath to breath consecutively. This will affect alveolar ventilation significantly. Figure 6-10 demonstrates the volume delivery changes that occur with changes in lung characteristics when using pressure-cycled ventilators.

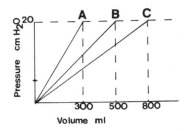

Fig. 6-10. Changes in volume delivery that occur with changes in lung characteristics when using pressure-cycled ventilators. *(A)* ↓ compliance or ↑ airway resistance. *(B)* Normal compliance and airway resistance. *(C)* ↑ compliance or ↓ airway resistance.

As with time-cycled ventilators, these changes in volume result in an inability to regulate alveolar ventilation. This phenomenon has resulted in a wide use of volume-cycled ventilators for assisted ventilation.

The third phase of a ventilator cycle is the expiratory phase. The expiratory phase is normally passive, resulting in lung pressure equilibrating with atmospheric pressure or zero end expiratory pressure (ZEEP) and the end of gas flow out of the lungs. Ventilators may have the capability to retard exhalation or maintain positive pressure during the entire expiratory phase. Expiratory retard is frequently used with chronic obstructive lung disease patients. Their airways may collapse early in the expiratory phase, thus promoting air trapping.

The objectives of PEEP are as follows:

1. ↑ Compliance
2. ↓ % shunt below 15%

Effects:

1. ↑ FRC
2. ↓ Closing volume
3. ↑ Pa_{O_2}
4. ↑ Oxygen transport

Adverse Effects:

1. Barotrauma
   a. Pneumothorax
   b. Pneumomediastinum
   c. Subcutaneous emphysema
2. ↓ Compliance
3. ↑ Pulmonary vascular resistance (PVR)
4. ↓ Cardiac output
5. ↑ Intracranial pressure

To increase compliance, the first indication for PEEP, we attempt to expand collapsed alveoli, thus resulting in a better ventilation perfusion match-up. As long as levels of compliance increase with the application of end expiratory pressure, overdistention of the alveoli to the point of increasing on PVR will not be a problem. Figure 6-11 represents the three stages alveoli go through with application of PEEP.

Going from a collapsed alveoli (*A*) to a normal expanded alveoli improves the FRC, compliance, closing volume, and % shunt without increasing PVR. This is considered "Best PEEP" or the best compliance level.

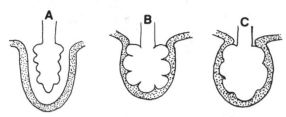

Fig. 6-11 (*A, B, C*). Three stages of alveoli with application of PEEP.

Collapsed	*Normal*	*Overdistention*
↓ FRC	FRC	↑ FRC
↓ Compliance	Compliance	↓ Compliance
↑ Closing vol.	Closing vol.	↓ Closing vol.
↑ % Shunt	Shunt	↓ % Shunt
↑ PVR	PVR	↑ PVR
↓ $\dot{V}/\dot{Q}$	$\dot{V}/\dot{Q} = 0.8$	↑ $\dot{V}/\dot{Q}$

Sometimes the best compliance level will not result in the best Pa_{O_2}, or a sufficient Pa_{O_2} level. It may be necessary to use higher levels of PEEP even though we know the compliance will decrease and PVR will increase when the best compliance level is exceeded. In these cases, the shunt is so bad it takes a higher level of PEEP to reduce it. Usually, a shunt above 15% will result in the need for higher levels of PEEP. The increased PVR results in a ↓ cardiac output (C.O.); but with I.V. therapy and vasopressors C.O. can be maintained. Thus, the % shunt will be reduced and O_2 transport can be maintained. This application of PEEP is known as optimal PEEP.

Some of the common abbreviations utilized in Phase III are NEEP, ZEEP, and PEEP.

NEEP: negative end-expiratory pressure

ZEEP: zero end-expiratory pressure

PEEP: positive end-expiratory pressure

Phase IV ends exhalation and begins inspiration. This can be facilitated by the patient or the machine itself, or by a combination of both. When a patient initiates inspiration, thus ending exhalation, he is said to be assisting the ventilator and thereby regulating his own respiratory rate. If the respiratory rate is exclusively controlled by the machine, the patient is said to be controlled. These "modes of ventilation" demonstrate patient

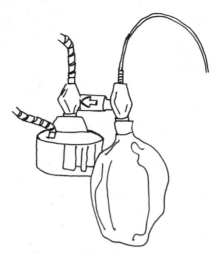

Fig. 6-12. IMV external set-up.

effort in terms of initiating inspiration. Volume can be regulated by the ventilator.

A third "mode of ventilation" exists, known as assitor-controller. A base rate is established on the ventilator, but the patient is allowed to initiate his own rate around the base rate established. This mode is a way of guaranteeing a minimum base rate for the patient in case of apnea.

Intermittent mandatory ventilation (IMV) is another mode of therapy which allows the patient to breathe spontaneously, but periodically an inspiratory cycle initiated by the ventilator gives a "mandatory" breath. The separate reservoir of gas from which the patient breathes spontaneously is sometimes incorporated in the ventilator, and sometimes externally applied to the ventilator. There are many advantages to IMV:

1. ↓ mean intrathoracic pressure.
2. Enhances the "Thoracic Pump."
3. Allows patient to regulate own Pa_{CO_2} level.
4. ↓ incidence of barotrauma.
5. Allows muscles of inspiration and exhalation to be utilized and coordinated.
6. Easier to wean patient from mechanically assisted ventilation.

Some ventilators are equipped with the ability to synchronize the control breath with the patient's spontaneous breathing. This prevents the control breath from the ventilator from cycling while a patient is in a spontaneous ventilatory cycle. The control breath will be delivered when the patient initiates the very next inspiration. This synchronizing ability is referred to as synchronized intermittent mandatory ventilation (SIMV).

With an understanding of the four phases every ventilator must pass through for a complete ventilatory cycle of inspiration and exhalation, it becomes appropriate to place ventilators available today within this classification system (Table 6-3). Table 6-4 lists the same ventilators with some of their capabilities. Understanding these capabilities aids in the proper selection of a ventilator for specific therapeutic needs such as PEEP, inspiratory plateau, large or small tidal volumes, etc.

With an understanding of the classification system and the various capabilities of specific ventilators, the respiratory clinician can make an educated selection of a ventilator for clinical use. The respiratory clinician should be able to select a ventilator which can accomplish the therapeutic needs outlined in a physician's order, which should include:

1. Mode of ventilation (*i.e.*, assist, control, assist-control, IMV or SIMV).

2. Tidal volume (usually between 10-15 ml./kg. of body weight).

3. Respiratory rate (usually between 10-15 breaths per minute).

4. Inspiratory/Expiratory ratio (usually 1/2).

5. Desired F_{IO_2} (begin with F_{IO_2} 0.9 until calculation for accurate F_{IO_2} can be made).

6. Sigh volume (1.5-2 × V_T).

7. Sigh frequency (at least every 5 minutes).

8. PEEP level, inspiratory plateau or expiratory resistance if desired.

It should be anticipated that some of the initial settings will have to be readjusted depending on each patient's response to the ventilator. Usually normal arterial blood gas levels (pH 7.35-7.45, Pa_{CO_2} 35-45, Pa_{O_2} 80-100) should be maintained as the guidelines for any ventilator adjustments.

With a physician's order secured, the respiratory clinician can begin the procedure which will result in the connection of the ventilator to the patient's artificial airway.

(*Text continues on p. 166.*)

Table 6-3. Classification of Specific Ventilators

Phase I				Phase II			Phase III			Phase IV					
Constant Flow Generator	Non-Constant Flow Generator	Pressure Generator	Inspiratory Plateau	Time-Cycled	Pressure Cycled	Volume-Cycled	ZEEP	PEEP	Expiratory Retard	Assistor	Controller	Assistor/Controller	IMV	SIMV	Ventilator
		X				X	X	X	X	X	X	X			Bennett MA-1
		X				X	X	X		X	X	X	X	X	Bennett MA-2
		X	X			X	X	X		X	X	X	X		Gill 1
X						X	X	X		X	X	X	X	X	Bourns Bear 1
X				X			X	X		X	X	X	X		Foregger 210
		X	X			X		X		X	X	X			Ohio 560
		X	X					X		X	X	X	X		Ohio CCV
X		X	X			X				X	X	X	X		Searle
X				X	X	X	X	X		X	X	X			Monaghan 225
	X			X			X	X			X				Emerson 3PV
	X			X			X	X			X		X		Emerson IMV
X				X				X		X	X	X	X		Veriflo CV 2000
X				X						X	X	X		X	Veriflo 200
	X		X	X				X	X		X				Engstrom ECS 2000
	X		X	X				X			X				Engstrom ER 300

Table 6-4. Capabilities of Ventilators

	TIDAL VOL. (ml.)	RATE (min.)	INSPIRATORY HOLD (sec.)	EXPIRATORY RETARD	PEEP (cm.H₂O)	PRESSURE LIMIT (cm.H₂O)	INSPIRATORY FLOW RATE (1 pm.)	O₂ CONTENT WATER %
Bennett MA-1	100-2200	6-60	NA	NA	0-20	10-80	15-100	21-100
Bennett MA-2	100-2200	0-60	0-2	NA	0-45	20-80	0-125	21-100
Gill	150-2100	6-60	0-2	NA	0-50	20-100	10-120	21-100
Bourns Bear 1	100-2000	0.5-60	0-2	NA	0-30	0-100	20-120	21-100
Foregger 210	80-8000	0.5-75	0.2-2	NA	0-35	20-110	12-120	21-100
OHIO 560	100-2000	6-60	0-2	NA	0-12	10-100	180	21-100
OHIO CCV	100-2000	5-40	0-2	NA	0-15	10-100	240	21-100
Searle VVA	300-2200	5-60	0-3	NA	0-20	10-100	20-200	21-100
Monaghan 225	100-3300	4-60	NA	NA	0-20	10-100	10-100	21-100
Emerson 3PV	20-2200	5-99	NA	NA	0-25	10-100	1.2-260	21-100
Emerson IMV	200-2200	0.2-22	NA	NA	0-25	50-100	5.5-60	21-100
Veriflo CV 2000	150-2000	8-60	NA	NA	0-20	20-100	12-100	21-100
Engstrom ECS 2000	20-1600	6-60		NA	0-20	10-100	0.2-384	21-100
Engstrom ER 300	20-2200	12-35	0-0.8	NA	0-20	30-90	1-264	21-100

CONNECTING VENTILATOR TO PATIENT

Description

Mechanical ventilation artificially supports the ventilation of a patient by providing volume, gas flow, and concentration at a rate which is physiologically sound.

Objectives

To maintain physiologic ventilation.
To manipulate ventilatory pattern and airway pressure.
· To decrease work of breathing.

Procedure

1. Secure physician's order for MAV.
2. Select appropriate ventilator.
3. Connect ventilator to various power sources, *e.g.*, electrical outlet, O_2 system.
4. Adjust sensitivity for "mode of ventilation," *e.g.*, assist, control, assist-control, IMV, SIMV.
5. Adjust T.V. (10-15 ml./kg.).
6. Adjust frequency to regulate Pa_{CO_2} as desired.
7. Adjust desired F_{IO_2} (initially F_{IO_2} 0.9).
8. Adjust inspiratory flow as necessary to achieve the desired I/E ratio.
9. Adjust sigh volume and frequency ($1.5\text{-}2 \times \dot{V}_T$ every 5 minutes).
10. Adjust pressure limits.
11. Using a test lung, manually cycle ventilator to insure it is functioning properly.
12. Connect ventilator circuit to patient's artificial airway.
13. Listen to patient's breath sounds, and watch for chest excursion when ventilator cycles into inspiratory phase.
14. Adjust low and high pressure alarms.
15. After 20 minutes obtain arterial blood gas sample.
16. Readjust T.V. or rate for desired pH and Pa_{CO_2}, and F_{IO_2} for desired Pa_{O_2}.

Special Considerations

• For the patient on continuous ventilation, a good humidifying system is necessary. Keep humidifier filled with sterile distilled water.
• Monitor F_{IO_2} and temperature on a continuous basis.

- Incorporate alarm systems that will alert you to high and low airway pressures and tidal volumes, power failure, etc.
- Never leave respirator patient unattended for any length of time.
- Monitor the patient's physiologic data frequently to assure that no complications are manifesting themselves (see Hazards).
- Obtain ABGs whenever ventilation parameters are changed.

Hazards

- Airway:
    - a. occlusion and obstruction of airway.
    - b. misplacement of airway (slipping into right mainstem bronchus).
    - c. high cuff pressure leading to necrosis and fistulas into the innominate artery and esophagus.
- Hypotension (high intrathoracic pressure):
    - a. ↓ cardiac output.
    - b. ↓ Cerebral blood flow.
    - c. ↓ renal blood flow.
    - d. ↓ tissue oxygenation.
- Atelectasis (repetitive T.V. without sighing):
    - a. ↓ FRC.
    - b. ↓ Compliance.
    - c. ↑ closing volume.
    - d. ↓ $\dot{V}/\dot{Q}$.
    - e. ↓ Pa_{O_2}.
- Pulmonary infection by cross-contamination.
- Gastrointestinal malfunction:
    - a. fecal impaction.
    - b. peptic ulcers.
- Barotrauma:
    - a. tension pneumothorax.
    - b. subcutaneous emphysema.
    - c. pneumomediastinum.
- Pulmonary:
    - a. increased $\dot{V}_D$.
    - b. ↑ pulmonary vascular resistance.
    - c. ↑ $\dot{V}/\dot{Q}$.
- Renal malfunction:
    - a. ↑ ADH (↓ right atrial pressure stimulation of pituitary gland).
    - b. ↓ renal blood flow (↓ cardiac output).

- An improperly trained, incompetent person can be disastrous in the clinical area.
- The respiratory clinicians, nurses and physicians must be able to recognize physiologic and clinical signs which indicate problems or potential problems, and, at the same time, have complete understanding of the mechanical ventilator assisting the patient. Anything less than this will result in improper patient care and management, and could lead to injury or death of patients.
- Equipment failure is easily controllable with a competent respiratory clinician. The common complications associated with equipment failure are outlined below:

1. Tubing system:
   a. disconnection between ventilator and patient.
   b. obstruction due to kinking or to H_2O which has condensed inside the tubing.
   c. fractures in the tubing leading to leaking of T.V.

2. Ventilator failure:
   a. electrical failure.
   b. pneumatic system failure.
   c. altered ventilator settings.

3. Humidification device:
   a. decrease water supply.
   b. too low or too high temperature.
   c. leaks in system.

4. Monitoring device failure:
   a. not activated.
   b. improperly adjusted.
   c. mechanical malfunction.

As stated previously, the respiratory clinician should be able to identify any of these complications.

Maintenance

- All tubing and humidifiers (patient circuit) must be exchanged daily.
- If tubing fills with condensate, empty water from circuit (not back into system).
- Change permanent filters every 500 hours.

BEST PEEP

Description

PEEP is a treatment modality used in conjunction with prolonged artificial ventilation. It keeps a positive pressure in the lungs even at end-expiration.

Objectives

To increase pulmonary compliance.
To decrease pulmonary shunt.

Procedure

1. Evaluate patient's vital signs (blood pressure, respiratory rate and heart rate).
2. Using inspiratory plateau or full expiratory resistance, obtain the equilibration pressure.
3. Divide the equilibration pressure into the exhaled volume to determine the patient's static compliance at ZEEP.
4. Add 3 cm.H_2O of PEEP (use the PEEP adjustment dial if available and register 3 cm.H_2O on the system pressure manometer or submerge 3 cm. of corrugated tubing under water and connect the opposite end to the exhalation manifold).
5. Repeat Steps 2 and 3.
6. If the static compliance has increased, add 3 cm.H_2O (total of 6 cm.H_2O PEEP).
7. Repeat Steps 2 and 3.
8. If the static compliance has decreased, reduce level of PEEP until the highest level of compliance can be achieved without resulting in a decrease.
9. Reevaluate vitals.
10. Obtain ABGs after 20 minutes.

Special Considerations

- If the best PEEP level does not provide a high enough Pa_{O_2}, then the physician must revert to higher levels of PEEP, which will compromise cardiac output. In that case, the goal must be to reduce the shunt level to below 15% and to maintain cardiac output with IV therapy and vasopressors.
- Monitor physiologic parameters to identify possible adverse effects.

- Assisted PEEP may be achieved by resetting the zero point for patient inspiratory effort.
- For determination of compliance, subtract PEEP level from plateau point to determine actual cm.H_2O. Divide by volume to find cm.H_2O/ml.

Hazards

- Decreased cardiac output
- Increased pulmonary vascular resistance
- Decreased compliance
- Pulmonary barotrauma
- Increased intracranial pressure

Maintenance

- System should be leak free in order to maintain a positive end pressure.

WEANING

Weaning the patient from the ventilator can usually be accomplished when the patient's physiologic parameters suggest that he/she can maintain adequate ventilation and oxygenation. It is extremely important that prior to any attempt to remove the patient from ventilatory assistance, the primary pathology be reversed, or under control with medication or some other therapy. As the pulmonary involvement is reversed, improvement of compliance, % shunt, airway resistance, inspiratory force and vital capacity will be noted.

Description

The systematic removal of a patient from MAV.

Objective

To assist the patient in the physiologic and psychological adjustment and the transition from mechanically assisted to spontaneous ventilation.

Procedure

If a patient meets the following physiologic parameters, then the weaning process probably can be initiated.

Table 6-5.
Physiologic Parameters That Indicate Ventilatory Weaning

Mechanics	Compliance	>30 ml./cm. H_2O
	Inspiratory force	>-25 cm. H_2O
	Vital capacity .	>14 ml./kg.
Ventilation	$\dot{V}_D/\dot{V}_T$	<0.55
	Pa_{CO_2}	35-45 mm. Hg
	pH	>7.35<7.45
Oxygenation	Pa_{O_2}	250-350 mm. Hg ($F_{I_{O_2}}$ = 1.0)
	% Shunt	< 15%

There are two common procedures for weaning patients from mechanically assisted ventilation.

The first is the use of IMV. As a patient's physiologic parameters improve, then less controlled breaths from the ventilator are needed, and thus the ventilator rate can gradually be decreased. This allows the patient to regulate his own Pa_{CO_2} and inspiratory effort. Eventually the burden of the entire ventilatory effort can be placed on the patient. When controlled breath rates are diminished to approximately 2 or 3 breaths per minute, the patient can probably be weaned entirely from the ventilator, extubated, and only need periodic deep breathing exercises and supplemental oxygen.

Procedure for IMV

1. Evaluate patient's physiologic status to determine if weaning is indicated (Table 6-5).

2. Adjust ventilator to IMV mode or SIMV mode. If internal IMV reservoir is not available, establish IMV reservoir externally (Fig. 6-12).

3. Reduce "control" breath rate to level that will provide for desired Pa_{CO_2}. Remember to consider spontaneous rate in ventilation total.

4. Continue to reduce IMV rate as tolerated by patient. (Patient's spontaneous effort should become more efficient and Pa_{CO_2} should stabilize to desired level.)

5. When IMV rate is reduced to 2-3 breaths/min., the patient can be removed from MAV.

The second weaning technique utilizes a "T" piece, oxygen and humidity from an efficient nebulizer. When a patient meets the physiologic parameters indicating weaning, tube O_2 and humidity replace the ventilator. The initial weaning period will vary with the status of various patients and may be as short as 5 to 10 minutes every hour. During the weaning period, pulse, blood pressure and respiratory rate should be monitored.

Procedure for T-tube Weaning

1. Evaluate patient's physiologic status to determine if weaning is indicated.

2. Remove patient from MAV and place on T-tube with heated high humidity and appropriate oxygenation for 5-10 min./hour as tolerated.

3. Monitor pulse, blood pressure, and respiratory rate. Increases in these parameters may indicate an unsuccessful weaning attempt.

Table 6-6 provides guidelines for reinstitution of MAV.

Table 6-6. Criteria for Reinstitution of MAV

Heart rate	> 110/min. or increase of 20/min.
Blood pressure	Rise or fall 20 mm.Hg systolic, 10 mm.Hg diastolic
Respiratory rate	> 35/min.

4. If the physiologic parameters being monitored during the weaning period are acceptable, the weaning period can be progressively increased.

5. The weaning period can be increased as tolerated to a maximum of 1 hour and 50 min. off of the ventilator per 2-hour period.

Special Considerations

• Weaning should not take place during hours of sleep. The patient needs his rest and the weaning process can be tiring.

• When the patient can tolerate being off of the ventilator and his ability to maintain an adequate airway is ensured, extubation can be accomplished.

• Most postop patients can be weaned quickly after the anesthesia has worn off.

Hazards

- Adverse changes in physiologic parameters.
- 'Dependency on ventilatory support.

Maintenance

- Give support and encouragement to the patient throughout the weaning period.

BIBLIOGRAPHY

Burton, G. G., Gee, G. N., and Hodgkin, J. G.: Respiratory Care: A Guide to Clinical Practice. Philadelphia, J. B. Lippincott Company, 1977.

Kirby, R. R., Downs, J. B., and Civetta, J. M.: High-level positive end-expiratory pressure (PEEP) in acute respiratory insufficiency. Chest, 67(2): 1975.

Pontoppidan, H., *et al*.: Acute Respiratory Failure in the Adult. Boston, Little, Brown and Co., 1973.

Shapiro, B. A., Harrison, R. A., and Trout, C. A.: Clinical Application of Respiratory Care. Chicago, Year Book Medical Publishers, Inc., 1975.

Sutter, P. M., Fairley, H. B., and Eisenberg, M. D.: Optimum end-expiratory airway pressure in patients with acute pulmonary failure. N. Eng. J. Med., 292(6): 1975.

CHAPTER SEVEN

Monitoring
Robert Fluck, B.S., R.R.T.

GENERAL CONSIDERATIONS FOR MONITORING

In monitoring a patient receiving respiratory therapy, we generally want the answers to three questions:

1. Are my equipment and its interface with the patient functioning correctly?

2. Are my ministrations having a beneficial effect on the patient?

3. Is the patient's condition improving or deteriorating?

To answer these, we must monitor, in any given situation, several of the following parameters:

$F_{I_{O_2}}$

Temperature

Exhaled volume

Airway pressure

Pulmonary mechanics

Lung volumes and flows

Cuff pressure

Arterial blood gases

Pulmonary hemodynamics

With this in mind, in this chapter we will discuss the equipment and procedures involved in obtaining the values for the above parameters. Normal values, accuracy, maintenance, special considerations, and advantages or disadvantages are shown, for rapid accessibility, on quick-reference charts.

OXYGEN ANALYZERS

Description

Analysis of $F_{I_{O_2}}$.

Objective

To insure accurate inspired gas mixture in order to permit proper assessment of patient's condition—an arterial blood gas is worthless unless the F_{IO_2} is accurately known.

Procedure

1. Check the meter zero of each of the hand-held analyzers prior to use.
2. Do not use if the meter cannot be zeroed.
3. Check each once daily for accuracy at F_{IO_2} of 1.0.
4. Prior to each use, check to insure a 0.21 reading on room air.
5. If there is a battery-check button, check the battery condition before each use.

Special Considerations

- The three hand-held analyzers read in partial pressure but have scales calibrated to F_{IO_2}, assuming a total pressure of 760 mm.Hg.
- If these are used at higher or lower elevations, the F_{IO_2} scale must be replaced with one using the total pressure at that altitude as F_{IO_2} 1.0.
- In an IMV circuit, if the ventilator and IMV flow are from different sources, each source should be analyzed separately.

Hazards

- With the exception of the Beckman D-2, none of the analyzers is safe for use in flammable atmospheres

Maintenance

- See Table 7-1.

TEMPERATURE INDICATORS

Description

Measures the temperature of the gas being inhaled by the patient.

(Text continues on p. 178.)

Table 7-1. Oxygen Analyzers

Type	Typical Brand & Model	Operation	Accuracy	Maintenance	Special Considerations
Polarographic Fig. 7-1	IL 413	Check battery with test button. Insert in line with adapter. Turn on and read with stand on a flat surface.	± 1%	Replace batteries when battery check indicates they are bad. Replace electrolyte and membrane periodically or when readings are erratic.	Not suitable for continuous monitoring as water on membrane will cause erratic readings.
Fuel cell Fig. 7-2	Harris-Lake; Teledyne	Is "ON" continuously. Using adapter provided, place in contact with gas to be monitored and read F_{IO_2}.	± 2%	Replace cell when readings become erratic (100,000 percent-hours is the useful life). Cell should last 6-9 months in normal use.	Easily damaged. Low cost.
Mass spectrometer Fig. 7-3	Perkin-Elmer	A membrane-tipped catheter is placed in an artery. The machine removes gas under vacuum to be analyzed.	±1%	Professional.	Very expensive. Very versatile. Can measure several gases in different patients sequentially.
Paramagnetic Fig. 7-4	Beckman D-2	Insert sample tubing into gas to be measured. Squeeze and release bulb 5-6 times (not necessary in ventilator circuit). Read on *flat* surface. If reading fluctuates from ventilator cycling, kink hose while reading.	± 2%	Replace batteries & bulb when they do not function. Replace silica gel when it turns pink.	High purchase and repair cost. Safe in flammable atmospheres. If placed on Healthdyne IMV controller, it will stop. Silica crystals should be blue. Halotnane will cause false high reading.

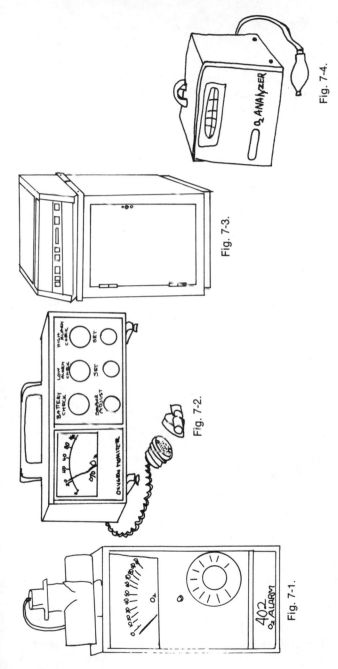

Fig. 7-1.

Fig. 7-2.

Fig. 7-3.

Fig. 7-4.

402
O₂ ALARM

OXYGEN MONITER

O₂

BATTERY CHECK   LOW ALARM CHECK   HIGH ALARM CHECK

ZERO ADJUST   SET   SET

O₂ ANAlyzer

Objective

To deliver the gas as close to body temperature saturated (37°C, 100% relative humidity) as possible in order to eliminate any water loss and drying of secretions in the patient.

Procedure

1. Place the device as close to the patient connection as possible as the gas cools about 1°C for each foot of tubing.
2. Check temperature each time ventilator is checked.

Special Considerations

• All devices should be periodically checked against a known standard for accuracy.

Hazards

• None with devices themselves; gas above body temperature can cause respiratory burns, gas below body temperature can cause drying of secretions with the attendant hazards.

Maintenance

• See Table 7-2.

SPIROMETERS

Description

Spirometers monitor or measure patient's tidal volume, forced vital capacity (FVC), and forced expiratory volume in one second (FEV_1).

Objectives

Monitoring the tidal volume, to insure the delivery to the patient of the desired volume. In measurement of FVC and FEV_1, to determine whether a patient can sustain his ventilation without mechanical assistance.

Procedure

1. For FEV_1 and FVC, see Table 7-6.
2. For exhaled volume, connect a monitoring spirometer (preferably with an alarm) to the expiratory line.

Table 7-2. Temperature Indicators

Type	Typical Brand	Advantages	Disadvantages
Liquid Crystal Fig. 7-5	Opti-temp	Rugged; accuracy-controlled during manufacture; can be placed very close to patient connection.	Color changes are hard to see in dim light.
Thermometer Fig. 7-6	Bennett Bunn	Low cost; most are easy to read.	Liquid can separate if instrument is jarred; in many cases must be placed in manifold, several feet away from patient connection.
Thermistor	Bennett Cascace II	Can be used as part of a feedback circuit to control heater output.	Needs complicated electronic circuit to be used.

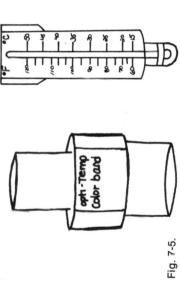

Fig. 7-5.

Fig. 7-6.

Table 7-3. Spirometers

Type	Typical Brand	Accuracy	Maintenance	Advantages/Disadvantages
Vortex Fig. 7-8	Bourns LS-75	± 5%	Remove ultrasonic transducer/detector and dry with alcohol pad if readings become erratic. Keep spare battery pack in charger and change each shift.	Display of volume to 1 ml. gives false sense of accuracy. Reads flow in either direction. Accurate from 5-250 l./min.
Vane Fig. 7-9	Wright	± 5% (assuming 15 l/min. minimal flow rate)	Use one-way valve assembly to prevent cross contamination (See Figure 7-7).	Easily damaged if dropped. Accurate only from 20-30 l./min. flow. May be damaged at flows over 200 l./min.
Volume Displacement Fig. 7-10	Bennett monitoring spirometer	± 50 ml	Remove water when it collects inside.	Most accurate: can accommodate an alarm; malfunctions easily corrected.

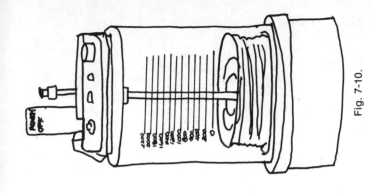

Fig. 7-10.

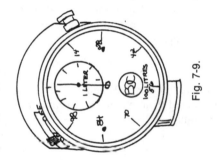

Fig. 7-9.

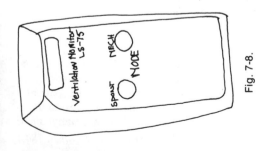

Fig. 7-8.

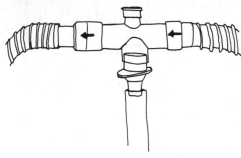

Fig. 7-7.

Special Considerations

• To prevent cross-contamination when measuring FVC and FEV₁, each patient should have his own one-way valve assembly (See Fig. 7-7). With this, the patient inhales room air and exhales into the spirometer.

Hazards

• A patient who is on an F_{IO_2} greater than 0.21 and/or PEEP may become hypoxic if disconnected from oxygen and ventilatory support for any period of time.

Maintenance

• See Table 7-3.

ALARMS

Description

An audible and visual indication of equipment malfunction or patient disconnection from equipment.

Objective

To insure that the patient is receiving the appropriate volume from a ventilator, to alert the therapist of a condition, such as accumulation of secretions, which has caused the patient's compliance to decrease, to insure the patient receives an accurate $F_{I_{O_2}}$, or to monitor I/E ratio and rate (as on a Baby Bird).

(Text continues on p. 184.)

Table 7-4. Alarms

Type	Typical Brand	Use	Advantages/Disadvantages
Volume	Bennett Spirometer Alarm	Adjusted with white stick to within 100 ml of consistently attained tidal volume. Change battery when alarm becomes soft.	Measures volume directly.
Pressure			
Low Only	Bunn LT 40 Bunn LT 50 Healthdyne	Pressure gradient (differential) adjusted so alarm senses about 10cm.H_2O below ventilator cycling pressure.	Healthdyne has no visual indication of when alarm is sensing pressure to aid in setting. Healthdyne uses batteries; Bunn 120 VAC.
High & Low	Bunn LT 60 Healthdyne	Bunn is set with selector switches in steps every 10cm.H_2O up to 50cm.H_2O (low) or 60cm.H_2O (high); Healthdyne must be set with continuous range knob.	Healthdyne uses batteries; Bunn 120 VAC. Bunn settings frequently several cm.H_2O off.
I:E Ratio	Healthdyne	Attached to circuit via small-bore tubing. I:E ratio, rate, and inspiratory or expiratory time can be displayed.	Only type available now.
O_2 Analyzer	Healthdyne	In-line adapter placed in circuit. High and low limits are set. Membrane is changed every six months or when readings become erratic. Battery checked daily with test button on back.	No moisture enters system to affect readings. Accuracy $\pm$ 1%. Uses polarographic principle.

Procedure

1. Attach the volume alarm to the expiratory line; another connection to the ventilator is needed to allow the spirometer to dump while the ventilator is in the inspiratory phase.

2. Connect pressure alarms to the patient circuit by a piece of small-bore tubing.

Special Considerations

- In patients with extremely high compliance, as in neuromuscular paralysis or in muscle atrophy, it may take a *lower* pressure to ventilate the patient than the low pressure alarm can be set for, and so a volume alarm is required.
- Set time delay to 15 seconds (or more, depending on respiratory rate) so patient can be suctioned or tubing emptied without setting off alarm.

Hazards

- All alarms are only as good as the person who resets them—the cause for the tripping of the alarm should be immediately determined.
- Also, excessive false tripping of alarms eventually causes people to ignore them.

Maintenance

- See Table 7-4.

PULMONARY MECHANICS

Description

Measurement and calculation of pulmonary parameters directly related to lung function and disease.

Objective

To assess patient's clinical condition, whether he is improving or deteriorating, and whether ministrations are actually helping him.

Procedure

See Table 7-5.

Special Considerations

- See Table 7-5.

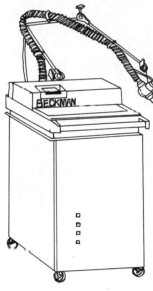

Fig. 7-11.

Hazards

• See Table 7-5.

BEDSIDE PULMONARY FUNCTION STUDIES

Description

Measurement of FVC and FEV_1.

Objective

To determine whether patient can adequately ventilate himself without assistance.

Procedure

See Table 7-6.

Special Considerations

• See discussion on spirometers.

Hazards

• See discussion on spirometers.

(Text continues on p. 191.)

Table 7-5. Pulmonary Mechanics

Name	Formula	Method	Comments
Compliance	$\dfrac{\text{Plateau pressure}}{\text{Exhaled tidal volume}}$	Using inspiratory hold (or temporarily occluding the exhalation valve), determine equilibration pressure. Divide by exhaled tidal volume.	Units: $1/\text{cm.H}_2\text{O}$, normal 0.1 Decreases in most disease entities. Used to determine best PEEP.
Resistance	$\dfrac{\text{Peak plateau pressure}}{\dfrac{\text{Tidal volume}}{\text{Inspiratory time}}}$	Subtract plateau pressure from peak cycling pressure. Divide by average inspiratory flow rate.	Units: $\text{cmH}_2\text{O}/\text{l./sec.}$ normal 0.6-2.4 @ .5/l./sec. Increases in some chronic diseases (asthma, bronchitis).
Intrapulmonary Shunt	$\dfrac{Cc_{O_2} - Ca_{O_2}}{Cc_{O_2} - C\overline{v}_{O_2}}$	Determine arterial content from arterial blood gas. Determine mixed venous content from pulmonary artery sample. For capillary content, assume $Pa_{O_2} = PA_{O_2}$ and calculate hemoglobin saturation and dissolved oxygen.	Units: Per cent, normal < 5 Used to determine optimal PEEP.
$\dot{V}_D : \dot{V}_T$ Ratio	Est. $\dfrac{Pa_{CO_2}}{40} \times \dfrac{\text{Actual } \dot{V}_E}{\text{Pred } \dot{V}_E} \times 0.33$ Meas. $\dfrac{Pa_{CO_2} - Pe_{CO_2}}{Pa_{CO_2}}$	For the estimate (which is quite close to the measured), use a Radford Nomogram for $\dot{V}_E$ (Est.), and measure $\dot{V}_E$. For the measured value, mean Pe_{CO_2} must be measured with a Capnograph.	Units: None. Normal 0.33 For weaning should be <0.55.
Vital Capacity	—	See section on bedside pulmonary function tests.	Units: ml. Normal - per chart. With inspiratory force is best indicator of ease of weaning. For weaning should be > 12 ml./kg.

Inspiratory Force	—	Use manometer (such as Boehringer inspiratory force gauge) with adapter on tracheal tube or mask on face. Use device with open port which can be manually occluded when force is measured and left open in between measurements.	Units: cm.H_2O. Normal > -70. For weaning, should be > -25.
A-VO_2 Difference	$CaO_2 - C\bar{V}O_2$	See shunt above.	Units: ml.O_2/100ml. blood. Normal 4-5. If increases, cardiac output is insufficent for tissue demands.

Table 7-6. Bedside Pulmonary Functions

Type	Procedure	Results
Forced Vital Capacity	Patient should have procedure explained before being placed on device. Nose clips should be placed on his nose and he should be instructed to seal his lips tightly around the mouthpiece. After about 1 minute of tidal ventilation to accustom him to the equipment, he should be instructed to take as deep a breath as possible, hold it for a short period and then exhale as hard as possible for as long as he can. This should be repeated 3 times and the best effort used in calculations. On a spirometer producing a recording (such as the Collins 7 Liter Survey (Spirometer) VC is the difference between the plateaus at top and bottom. Procedure for electronic spirometers (such as Monaghan, Donti, or LSE) may differ slightly.	Use predicted normal from a nomogram (such as Cory). If value is ± 20% of predicted it is considered WNL. Decreased values appear in restrictive disease with normal $FEV_1/FVC\%$ and in obstructive disease with decreased $FEV_1/FVC\%$.
$\dfrac{FEV_1 \%}{FVC}$	Using the time markings on the graph paper, one should determine one second. Measuring the volume from the peak inspiratory plateau to the one second point will give FEV_1. Divide this by the FVC measured above and express as a per cent.	Using actual FEV_1 and FVC, normal for 20-year-old male is 83% and decreases approximately 2% for every 10 years. Although there are tables for normal FEV_1, they are essentially worthless as they are not related to FVC. For example, if the FVC is decreased, the FEV_1 will certainly be decreased, but as a per cent of FVC may be normal. The value is a gross indicator of airways obstruction.

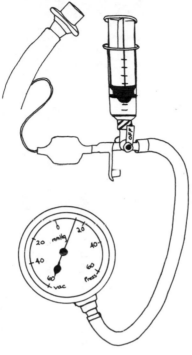

Fig. 7-12.

CUFF PRESSURE MEASUREMENT

Description

Determination of pressure exerted by tracheal tube cuff on wall of trachea.

Objective

To maintain pressure on the wall of the trachea under 20 mm. Hg, allowing capillary blood flow and preventing tissue necrosis.

Procedure

See Table 7-7. There are basically three types of cuff designs on the market: the Lanz, the Kamen-Wilkinson, and "all the rest" (made by manufacturers such as Portex and National

Table 7-7. Cuff Pressure Determination

Type	Procedure	Comments
Lanz	Not necessary—pressure in cuff is automatically limited to 20-25mm.Hg by valve.	Probably best type of cuff available.
"All The Rest" (See text) Fig. 7-12	The stopcock is plugged into the pilot tube. Once minimal-occluding volume (MOV, no-leak) or minimal leak (ML) has been established, stopcock is turned to allow manometer to be connected to cuff and pressure is read.	Should be done at least twice per shift.
Kamen-Wilkinson Fig. 7-13	Once tube has been inserted, all air is withdrawn with a syringe; the pilot port is clamped and the syringe is released. Using the volume in ml. the pressure on the trachea is read off the graph.	Pilot cuff must *never* be corked if cuff is to retain low pressure characteristics. May leak slightly at cycling pressures over 40cm.H_2O.

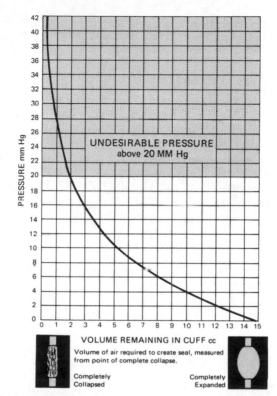

VOLUME REMAINING IN CUFF cc

Volume of air required to create seal, measured from point of complete collapse.

Completely Collapsed

Completely Expanded

HOW TO USE THE KAMEN-WILKINSON PRESSURE CHART

- After intubation and a seal has been effected insert the syringe into the open pilot port and extract ALL of the air to a negative force.

- Clamp the pilot port (not the pilot tube) with fingers or hemostat and release the plunger of the syringe.

- The plunger will come to rest on a reading of cc's of air. This reading is the volume of air remaining in the cuff at the point of seal, measured from the point of complete collapse.

- Remove the syringe and leave pilot port open. This will reseal the trachea.

- Refer to pressure graph. Pressure reading is at the point that the volume line intersects the curve. Pressures of 20mm Hg. or more are considered undesirable.

Example:

If 5 cc's of air can be extracted from the cuff after it has sealed (i.e. volume of air remaining in cuff) the lateral wall pressure is 11mm Hg.

* This pressure chart was formulated with a No. 6 trach tube. Larger size cuffs have a residual volume up to 24cc. In these, the pressure curve has a similar contour but intersects the 20mm Hg. line at 5 or 6cc.

Fig. 7-13.

Catheter Corporation). The Lanz needs no check on pressure. The Kamen-Wilkinson uses a unique method to estimate pressure (Table 7-7). The cuff pressure in the rest of the tubes, regardless of design differences, is measured in the same manner.

Special Considerations

- If the pilot tube on a Kamen-Wilkinson tube is accidentally removed, the cuff can still be deflated by cutting off the tip of a 19- or 20-gauge needle and inserting it into the pilot tube.
- If the pilot tube is torn completely off, a 19- or 18-gauge needle with the tip cut off can be inserted into the hole and the cuff deflated in this way.
- See Table 7-7 for additional considerations.

Hazards

- Cuff may become partially deflated, allowing secretions to enter trachea.
- High cuff pressure can result in necrosis, fibrosis and, ultimately, tracheal stenosis, a severe complication.

SWAN-GANZ CATHETER

Description

Obtains hemodynamic and blood gas data from the low-pressure side of the circulation.

Objective

To assess accurately the patient's cardiopulmonary status.

Procedure

See Table 7-8.

Special Considerations

- Catheter may need to be inserted by a physician, depending on institutional procedure.
- *Any* patient on greater than 10cm.H_2O PEEP should have a Swan-Ganz catheter and an arterial line inserted.

Table 7-8. Swan-Ganz Catheter

Function	Procedure	Normal	Comments
Pulmonary Artery Pressure	Continuously monitored on oscilloscope (CRT Screen) for hemodynamics; diastolic (PAD) can be close to LA pressure (but is not always). Mean pressure used for calculating pulmonary vascular resistance.	25/10-12 mean 15-18mm.Hg PVR 150-250 dyne cm./sec.[5]	PVR is calculated as $\dfrac{\text{pressure}}{\text{flow}}$. If units of mm.Hg/L./min. are used, normal is 1.5-2.0. If mm.Hg/ml./sec. are used, normal is 0.1.
Left Atrial (LA) Pressure	Balloon at tip of catheter is inflated (volume is stated on port for syringe) for less than one minute. Waveform should change to LA. Mean pressure is read.	5-10mm.Hg. mean	Abbreviations include PAW, PCW, PAo.
Central Venous Pressure	Monitored on oscilloscope or water manometer. Height of manometer or transducer for oscilloscope is vital—should be at level of right atrium.	0-5mm.Hg.	It is useful to mark a line on the side of the chest so that each reading is made at the same level.
Cardiac Output	Following instructions with cardiac output computer (made by KMA, Edwards Labs, and Instrumentation Labs), push start button and rapidly inject 10 ml. saline (0°C or 21°C, depending on machine).	Minimum 2.5 L./min./M² Cardiac index = $\dfrac{\text{C.O.}}{\text{B.S.A.}}$	Can be repeated every minute if necessary. Runs 7% higher than Fick but provides reproducible results.
A-V Oxygen Content Difference	See "Pulmonary Mechanics."	4-5 vol %	
Intrapulmonary shunt	See "Pulmonary Mechanics."	< 5%	

Hazards

• Those associated with any intravascular catheter, including thromboembolism and phlebitis, plus iatrogenic pulmonary infarct, rupture of chordae tendinae, and arrhythmias.

ARTERIAL PUNCTURE

Description

Arterial puncture is a method by which an arterial sample may be obtained.

Objective

To obtain arterial blood for blood gas analysis.

Procedure

1. Assemble equipment necessary for arterial puncture: glass or plastic syringe with free flowing barrel, prep pads, sterile gauze, sodium heparin, cork or rubber stopper, clear hub, short bevel needles (#20-#25 gauge), container with ice, label.
2. Approach the patient and explain the procedure.
3. Carefully select the puncture site. Check for collateral circulation by using the Allen Test if the radial artery is chosen.
4. Prepare the syringe.
   a. Heparinize syringe and needle.
   b. Remove air from syringe.
   c. Replace cap on needle.
5. Prepare the puncture area and your own fingers with prep pads.
6. Palpate the puncture site very carefully, using a two-finger method.
7. Penetrate the artery with the needle at a 45° angle and the bevel facing the flow of blood.
8. Watch for a flash of blood into the hub of the needle.
9. Hold the needle inside of the artery until the syringe fills to the desired level.
10. Apply firm pressure with sterile gauze, remove needle from artery, and continue to maintain pressure for 5 minutes.
11. Remove any air bubbles from the syringe.
12. Stick the end of the syringe into stopper immediately.
13. Mix sample well.

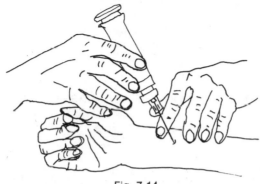

Fig. 7-14.

14. Label syringe with patient's name, date and time.
15. Place syringe in ice water bath.
16. Analyze immediately.

Special Considerations

- The radial artery is the artery of choice, followed by the brachial and femoral.
- Always check for collateral circulation with radial artery.
- Compress the artery for at least 5 minutes following the puncture.
- Sample should be analyzed within twenty minutes.
- For patients on anticoagulent therapy or history of bleeding disorder, compression of the artery may take an extended period of time.
- For patients with arteriosclerotic disease, compress artery only until bleeding stops.

Hazards

- Bleeding for patient on anticoagulent therapy or with Hx of bleeding.
- Hematoma.
- Nerve spasm.
- Severing of the artery.
- Arteriospasm.
- Infection.
- Thrombosis.
- Loss of limb.

Maintenance

- Examine the artery 5 minutes and 10 minutes after puncture to check for bleeding and complications.

INTERPRETATION OF ACID-BASE STATUS

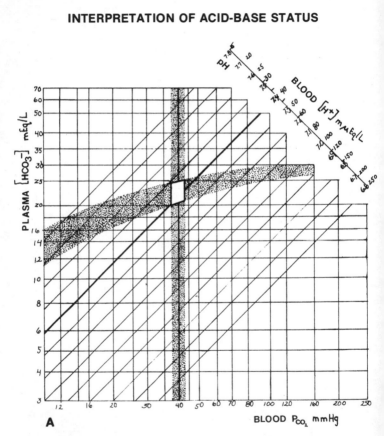

Fig. 7-15. Interpretation graphs and key. Plot Pa_{CO_2} and pH points on graph *A*. The interpretation point is the intersection of these 2 points. Find that point on graph *B*. Read the corresponding number and find its interpretation in *C*. To find plasma $[HCO_3^-]$, locate Pa_{CO_2} and pH on *A*. From that point, draw a line parallel to the Pa_{CO_2} axis. The intersection of this line with the $[HCO_3^-]$ axis indicates $[HCO_3^-]$ value. Note: pH falls 0.015 for each °C patient temperature rise. (Courtesy: John Mathoefer, M.D.)

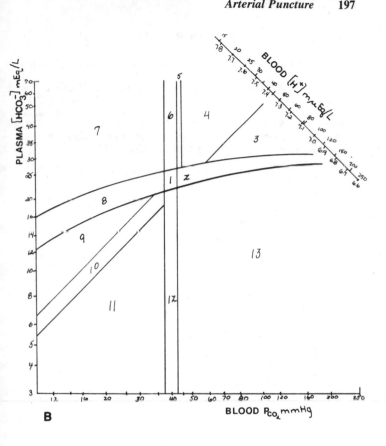

B

INTERPRETATION

1. Normal
2. Respiratory acidosis
3. Respiratory acidosis — compensated
4. Respiratory acidosis & metabolic alkalosis
5. Metabolic alkalosis — compensated
6. Metabolic alkalosis
7. Respiratory alkalosis & metabolic alkalosis
8. Respiratory alkalosis
9. Respiratory alkalosis — compensated
10. Metabolic acidosis & respiratory alkalosis
11. Metabolic acidosis — compensated
12. Metabolic acidosis
13. Metabolic acidosis & respiratory acidosis

C

BIBLIOGRAPHY

Levesque, P. R., and Rosenberg, H.: Rapid bedside estimation of wasted ventilation ($\dot{V}_D/\dot{V}_T$). Anesthesiology, *42*(1), 1975.

Shapiro, B. A., Harrison, R. A., and Walton, J. R.: Clinical Application of Blood Gases. Chicago, Year Book Medical Publishers, 1977.

Schroeder, J., and Daily, E.: Techniques in Bedside Hemodynamic Monitoring. St. Louis, C. V. Mosby Co., 1976.

Wernerus, H., Silva, G., and Wanner, A.: Accuracy of Drager & Wright ventilation meters. Respiratory Care, *23*:856, 1978.

CHAPTER EIGHT

Infection Control
Diane Blodgett, R.R.T.

GENERAL CONSIDERATIONS FOR INFECTION CONTROL

This section deals with the procedures for infection control, cleaning and decontamination, and bacteriological surveillance of respiratory therapy equipment.

If we perform all the other elements of respiratory care correctly and neglect the infection control measures and the bacteriological monitoring of our equipment, we are performing our duties for naught.

For respiratory therapy personnel, infection control measures should include an aseptic handwashing procedure, aseptic handling of supplies and equipment, and strict adherence to the principles of isolation. All of these procedures are included in this section.

Respiratory therapy equipment can provide a primary source of nosocomial infections. Therefore, infection control measures for equipment should include the use of filters, disposables, where appropriate, and the decontamination or sterilization of all permanent equipment.

The various methods of cleaning and decontamination of RT equipment are summarized here in a comparison chart (Table 8-1). Different methods produce varying results; cleaning merely removes organic or inorganic material, while a decontamination removes all pathogens. Sterilization means destruction of all microorganisms.

Whatever process is followed, certain guidelines should be adhered to. The dirty equipment should be in one area, clean in another, and the process should flow from dirty (contaminated) to clean (decontaminated). The surfaces of large pieces of

(Text continues on p. 202.)

Table 8-1. Methods of Cleaning and Decontamination

Method	Characteristics of Process	Advantages	Disadvantages	Equipment to be Decontaminated
Dry Heat (sterilization)	Very high temperatures. Low moisture content.	No toxic by-products. Inexpensive.	Damages heat sensitive equipment. Equipment cannot be identified through packaging. May have incomplete kill on short cycle.	Equipment that cannot be disassembled. Moisture sensitive equipment.
Steam Autoclaving (sterilization)	High temperatures. High moisture content. High pressures.	No toxic by-products. Completely kills all microorganisms including spores. Inexpensive, fast.	Damages heat and moisture sensitive equipment. Equipment cannot be identified through some packaging.	Surgical instruments. Linen. Some high density plastics.
Ethylene Oxide (sterilization)	Low temperature. ETO and carrier gas (Freon) necessary. Specific time, conc., tem., etc. must be adhered to.	Completely kills all microorganisms. Low temperature. Visibility of equipment through plastic wrap.	Expensive, time consuming. Must completely dry and clean equipment first. Aeration necessary to remove toxic by-products.	Plastics. Rubber. Respirators. All items heat or moisture sensitive.
Chemical Sterilization (decontamination or sterilization) Potentiated acid glutaraldehyde	Low pH liquid.	Room temperature. Lasts 4 weeks. Fast, sterilizes in 1 hour at 60° C (10 minutes for disinfection).	Somewhat expensive, not appropriate for most electrical equipment. Can cause contact dermititis in users. When equipment is improperly rinsed, toxic effect can result (burns). Possible recontamination during processing.	Plastics. Rubber. Metal.
Aqueous buffered glutaraldehyde	High pH liquid. Must be buffered to become activated.	Room temperature. Lasts two weeks. Fast, sterilizes in 10 hours.		

Pasteurization (decontamination)	Hot water immersion.	Relatively fast. Easy. No toxic by-products.	Expensive initial outlay. Recontamination can occur during processing. Not appropriate for electrical equipment or respirators. Heat damage.	Rubber. Plastics. Glass.
Ultrasonic (decontamination)	Sound waves pass through fluid vibrating which causes cleansing action.	Fast. Easy. Uses water as fluid.	Recontamination can occur during processing. Expensive initial outlay.	Rubber. Plastics. Surgical instruments. Glass.
Acetic Acid (specific decontamination)	Low pH liquid.	Inexpensive, for home use.	Smell. May be ineffective against most microorganisms.	Home care equipment.

equipment should be cleaned, then wiped down with a decontaminating agent. When the decontamination process is complete for smaller items, the package should include information on the type of process used, the initials of the therapist processing the equipment, the date of the processing and the date of expiration. This information allows the handling of that equipment to be traced in case a problem is encountered.

Monitoring our methods of decontamination or sterilization not only assures quality control, but also provides us with the reassurance that we are protecting the patient. It is most appropriate to test the effluent gas because this gas is what comes in contact with the patient. However, swabbing and rinse sampling may be appropriate in some cases. A regular (weekly) program of surveillance should include testing of both clean and used equipment. To double check your method of surveillance and your decontamination and/or sterilization procedures, periodically allow a piece of equipment to become contaminated, take a bacteriological sample, process the equipment, and take another sample.

ETHYLENE OXIDE STERILIZATION

Description

Ethylene oxide (ETO) sterilization brings about the destruction of microorganisms by the use of ETO gas at a certain relative humidity (50%), temperature (120-135°), concentration (12%), vacuum (25-27 inches) and time (3-4 hours). The microorganisms are killed by preventing their reproduction.

Objective

To kill all microorganisms present on equipment that is heat- and/or moisture-sensitive (*e.g.,* plastics, rubber, respirators).

Procedure

1. Disassemble equipment to be cleaned.
2. Clean equipment of all organic material.
3. Rinse equipment thoroughly to remove all cleanser residue.
4. Dry equipment *completely*.
5. Reassemble equipment in desired configuration.

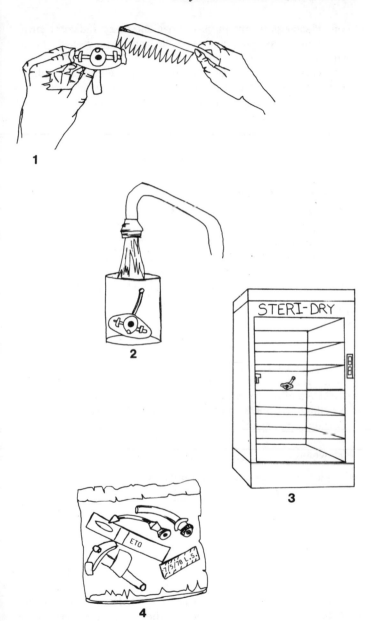

Fig. 8-1. ETO sterilization.

6. Place equipment in plastic bag and insert indicator strip.

7. Remove as much air as possible from bag and seal bag with heat sealer, twist tie or tape.

8. Place ETO tape on bag and mark package with date, expiration date, sterilization method and technician's name.

9. Stack packages in ETO sterilizer chamber.

10. Follow manufacturer's instructions for ETO cycle.

11. When cycle is complete, remove from chamber and aerate either on shelf or in an aeration chamber.

12. Store in clean area.

Special Considerations

• Equipment *must* be clean and dry before being packaged.
• Complete aeration must be assured—1 week on the shelf and 24 hours in aeration chamber.
• Plastic bags must be permeable to ETO.
• All sterilizing parameters (time, temperature, humidity, ETO concentration, and exposure time) must be met.

Hazards

• If equipment is not dry, water combines with ETO to form the toxic by-product etheylene glycol.
• Ethylene chorohydrin, a toxic by-product, may be formed when rubber is processed.
• Because of the by-products, skin irritation, laryngeal edema, swelling and burns may occur with improperly processed or aerated equipment.

Maintenance

• Shelf life for a tied or taped plastic package is 3 months; for a heat-sealed plastic package it is 1 year.

DRY HEAT

Description

Dry heat autoclaving is a sterilization technique that brings about the destruction of microorganisms by very high temperatures over a long period of time (1-6 hours). The microorganisms are destroyed by the disruption of their cell membrane and/or coagulation of the protoplasm.

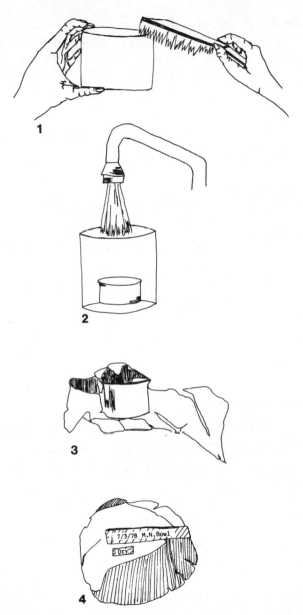

Fig. 8-2. Dry heat sterilization.

Objective

To kill all microorganisms present on equipment that can tolerate very high temperatures but cannot tolerate moisture, *e.g.,* moisture-sensitive equipment, equipment that cannot be disassembled.

Procedure

1. Disassemble equipment to be cleaned.
2. Clean equipment of all organic material.
3. Rinse equipment thoroughly to remove all cleanser residue.
4. Reassemble equipment in desired configuration.
5. Wrap equipment in porous towel or wrap.
6. Close wrap with indicator tape.
7. Wrap again with second towel or wrap unless a plastic/paper pouch is used.
8. Close wrap with indicator tape (heat seal pouch, if used) and mark package with expiration date, sterilization method and technician's name.
9. Stack packages in chamber of autoclave.
10. Follow manufacturer's instructions for dry heat cycle.
11. Remove from chamber following completion of cycle.
12. Store in clean area.

Special Considerations

- Use where steam is unavailable.
- Plastics will melt.
- Do not use this method for electrical equipment.
- After processing packs must remain dry to insure sterility.
- Rubber may deteriorate.

Hazards

- Burns may occur through careless handling of packs.

Maintenance

- Shelf life for cloth or paper wrap is 30 days; for plastic/paper pouch it is 90 days.

COLD CHEMICAL STERILIZATION

Description

Cold chemical sterilization is a decontamination or sterilization technique that brings about the destruction of all microorganisms, including spore, in one hour (potentiated acid gluteraldehyde) to 10 hours (aqueous buffered gluteraldehyde); these two products are bactericidal in 10-20 minutes. This technique requires the immersion of the equipment in the sterilization liquid. Microorganisms are destroyed by protein denaturation or enzyme degradation.

Objective

To decontaminate or sterilize equipment that can tolerate immersion in a liquid at room temperature or slightly elevated temperatures, *e.g.,* plastics, rubber, metal.

Procedure

1. Disassemble the equipment to be cleaned.
2. Set aside equipment that cannot be immersed.
3. Clean equipment of all organic material.
4. Rinse equipment thoroughly to remove all cleanser residue.
5. Remove excess water.
6. Immerse equipment in cold sterilizing liquid for the required length of time. (10-20 minutes for decontamination, 1-10 hours for sterilization). See Table 8-1.
7. Remove equipment from liquid.
8. Rinse thoroughly with sterile distilled water.
9. Dry completely in clean area.
10. Reassemble equipment.
11. Place equipment in plastic bag.
12. Seal bag with heat sealer, twist tie or tape.
13. Mark package with date, expiration date, decontamination method and technician's name.
14. Store in clean area.

Special Considerations

- Equipment *must* be clean before immersion in liquid.
- Completely immerse equipment in liquid; all surface areas must be in contact with liquid.

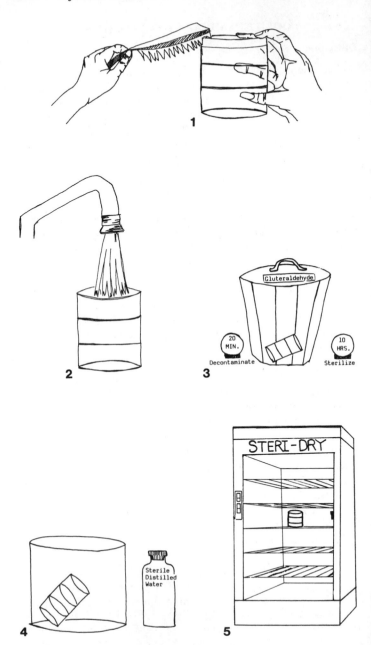

1

2

3

4

5

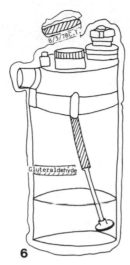

Fig. 8-3. Chemical decontamination.

- To prevent a contact dermititis, use gloves when handling liquid.
- Rinse equipment completely before drying to remove toxic residue.
- Possible recontamination can occur during processing. Following processing, handle equipment with sterile technique.
- Equipment must be completely dry before repackaging.

Hazards

- Contact dermititis.
- Recontamination.
- Toxic effects to patient when equipment is inadequately rinsed.

Maintenance

- Shelf life of 3 months.

STEAM AUTOCLAVE

Description

Steam autoclaving is a sterilization technique that brings about the destruction of microorganisms by steam under high tempera-

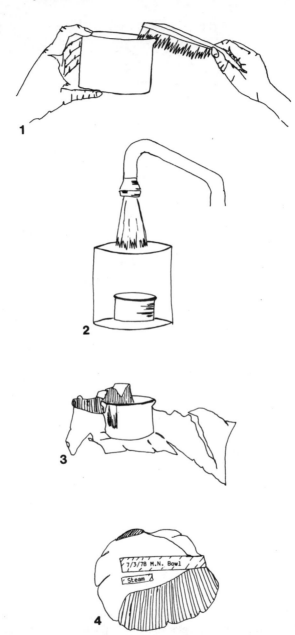

Fig. 8-4. Steam autoclaving.

ture and pressure. The microorganisms are destroyed by the disruption of the cell membrane and/or the coagulation of the cell protoplasm.

Objective

To kill all microorganisms present on equipment that can tolerate moisture and high temperatures, *e.g.,* linen, surgical packs, utensils.

Procedure

1. Disassemble equipment to be cleaned.
2. Clean equipment of all organic material.
3. Rinse equipment thoroughly to remove all cleanser residue.
4. Reassemble equipment in desired configuration.
5. Wrap equipment in porous towel or steam wrap. Include sterilization indicator strip.
6. Close wrap with indicator tape.
7. Wrap again with second towel or wrap, unless plastic/paper pouch is used.
8. Close wrap with indicator tape (heat seal pouch, if used) and mark with date, expiration date, sterilization method, and technician's name.
9. Stack packages to be steam autoclaved in steam chamber.
10. Follow manufacturer's instructions for steam cycle.
11. Remove from chamber following completion of cycle.
12. Store in clean area.

Special Considerations

- Electrical equipment can be harmed with this procedure.
- Plastics may melt.
- Rubber may deteriorate.
- Packs must remain dry to insure sterility, indicator tape will change from light to dark.

Hazards

- Burns may occur through careless handling of equipment.

Maintenance

- Shelf life for cloth wrap is 30 days, for paper wrap is 30-60 days, and for plastic/paper pouch is 90 days.

PASTEURIZATION

Description

Pasteurization is a decontamination technique that brings about the destruction of most microorganisms (except spores) by immersion of equipment in a hot (170°F) water bath for one hour. The microorganisms are destroyed by the heat coagulation of the cell protoplasm.

Objective

To decontaminate equipment that can tolerate heat and immersion in a liquid, *e.g.,* plastics, rubber.

Procedure

1. Disassemble equipment.
2. Set aside equipment that cannot be immersed.
3. Clean equipment of all orgnaic material.
4. Place equipment in pasteurizing water bath.
5. Immerse equipment for one hour.
6. Remove equipment from water bath.
7. Dry completely in clean area.
8. Reassemble equipment.
9. Place equipment in plastic bag.
10. Seal bag with heat sealer, twist tie or tape.
11. Mark package with date, expiration date, decontamination method and technician's name.
12. Store in clean area.

Special Considerations

- Equipment *must* be clean before immersion in water bath.
- Equipment must be completely dry before packaging.
- Possible recontamination can occur during processing. Following processing, handle equipment with sterile technique.

Hazards

- Burns can occur during processing.
- Recontamination.

Maintenance

- Shelf life of 3 months.

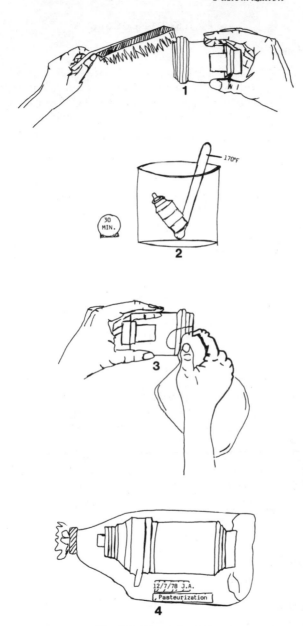

Fig. 8-5. Pasteurization.

ULTRASONIC CLEANER

Description

Ultrasonic cleaner is a decontamination technique that brings about the destruction of most microorganisms by the immersion of equipment in a liquid and the vibration of that liquid at a high frequency. The microorganisms are destroyed by disruption of cell membrane.

Objective

To decontaminate equipment that can tolerate immersion in a liquid at room temperature, *e.g.,* plastics, metal instruments.

Procedure

1. Disassemble equipment.
2. Set aside equipment that cannot be immersed.
3. Place equipment in ultrasonic cleaner.
4. Make sure distilled water covers equipment.
5. Add small amount of ultrasonic cleaner detergent.
6. Turn on ultrasonic cleaner.
7. Process equipment for 30 minutes.
8. Remove equipment from ultrasonic cleaner.
9. Dry completely in clean area.
10. Reassemble equipment.
11. Place equipment in plastic bag.
12. Seal bag with heat sealer, twist tie or tape.
13. Mark package with date, expiration date, decontamination method, and technician's name.
14. Store in clean area.

Special Considerations

• Possible recontamination can occur during processing. Following processing, handle equipment with sterile technique.
• Equipment must be completely dry before packaging.

Hazards

• Recontamination.

Maintenance

• Shelf life of 3 months.

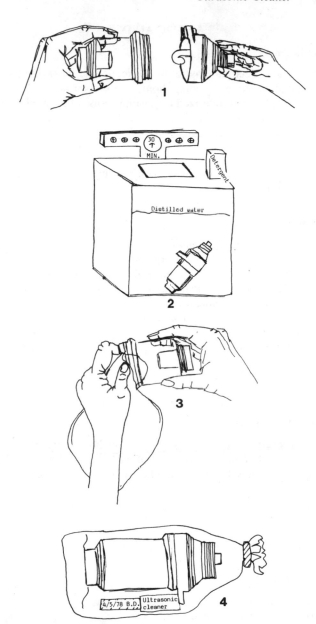

Fig. 8-6. Ultrasonic cleaner.

ACETIC ACID

Description

Acetic acid decontamination is the technique most often recommended to patients going home with respiratory therapy equipment. It is characterized by the immersion of the equipment. in a weak acetic acid solution.

Objectives

To decontaminate home care equipment for the respiratory therapy patient.

Procedure

1. Disassemble equipment.
2. Clean equipment of all organic material.
3. Rinse thoroughly to remove all cleaner residue.
4. Immerse equipment in acetic acid solution (0.25%).
5. Let soak 20 minutes.
6. Remove equipment from acetic acid.
7. Rinse thoroughly.
8. Dry completely in clean area.
9. Reassemble equipment.
10. Place equipment in plastic bag.
11. Store in clean area.

Special Considerations

- This procedure should only be used for home care patients.
- This should be done at the end of each day of therapy.
- Equipment may become recontaminated during processing.

Hazards

- Recontamination.
- Lacks effectiveness against most bacteria.

Maintenance

- New solution of acetic acid used each day.
- Process equipment each day.
- Shelf life of one day.

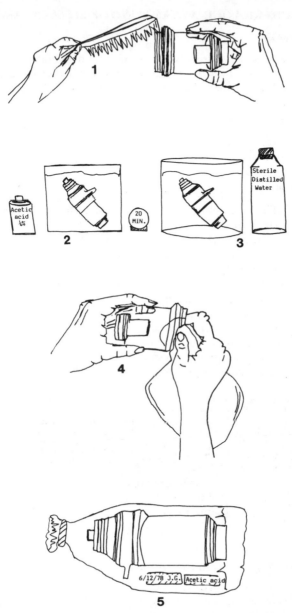

Fig. 8-7. Acetic acid.

BACTERIOLOGICAL SAMPLING OF EFFLUENT GAS

Description

This method of testing RT equipment for possible contamination uses a direct sample of the effluent gas over and/or through bacteriologic media.

Objective

To detect contamination of aerosol or humidity-producing respiratory therapy equipment.

Procedure

1. Obtain sampling equipment (Agar plates with sampling funnel attached).
2. Start machine, humidity- or aerosol-producing device.
3. Set device so that the maximum aerosol is being produced.
4. Allow equipment to run for at least 10 seconds.
5. Remove lid from sampling plate.
6. Insert hose into diverting funnel.
7. Sample effluent gas for 10 seconds.
8. Remove tubing from funnel.
9. Remove funnel and replace lid on plate.
10. Mark plate with identification data.
11. Send culture to lab or incubate for 24-48 hours at 37°C.

Special Considerations

• Remove mouthpieces or adaptors from respiration circuits before testing.
• If more than 20 colonies are recovered, the level of contamination is unacceptable.
• Handle plates with care to avoid contamination.
• Mark each plate for positive identification.
• Refer to manufacturer's guidelines for flow and rate settings.

Hazards

• Spread of pathogenic organisms.

Maintenance

• Commercial samplers may become outdated.

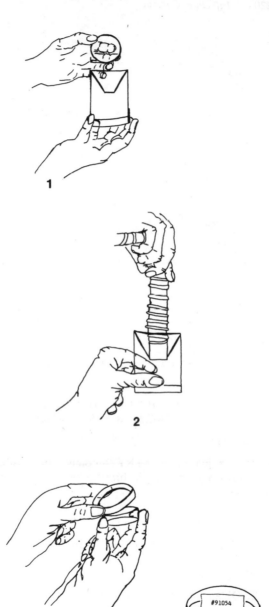

1

2

3

#91054

Fig. 8-8. Bacteriological sampling—effluent gas.

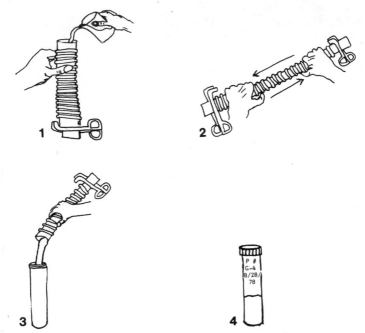

Fig. 8-9. Bacteriological sampling—broth rinse.

BACTERIOLOGICAL SAMPLING BY BROTH RINSE METHOD

Description

This method of testing RT equipment for possible contamination uses a bacteriologic broth which rinses through the RT equipment.

Objective

To detect contamination of Respiratory therapy equipment.

Procedure

1. Obtain sampling equipment (nutrient broth, sterile tube or flask, clamps).

2. For tubing, while holding tubing at each end, rinse some of broth through by raising and lowering each end alternately 50

times. For containers, add rinse broth to container, close off opening and shake vigorously for at least 30 seconds.

   3. Empty broth into sterile tube or flask.

   4. Mark tube or flask with identification data.

   5. Send culture to lab or incubate for 24-48 hours at 37°C.

Special Considerations

- Handle samples with care to avoid contamination.
- Clamps can be used to seal end of flexible tubing.
- Small containers may be immersed in broth, which is then cultured.
- Mark each sample for positive identification.
- If more than 20 colonies are recovered, the level of contamination is unacceptable.

Hazards

- Spread of pathogenic organisms.

Maintenance

- Use only currently dated supplies.

BACTERIOLOGICAL SAMPLING BY SWAB TECHNIQUE

Description

   This method of testing RT equipment for possible contamination uses a swab to sample the surface of the equipment.

Objective

   To detect contamination of respiratory therapy equipment.

Procedure

   1. Obtain sampling equipment (sterile swab, sterile saline, and nutrient broth in screw cap tube).

   2. Moisten swab with sterile saline.

   3. Apply to the area to be sampled.

   4. Immerse swab specimen in broth in the screw cap tube.

   5. Wring out swab and remove from tube.

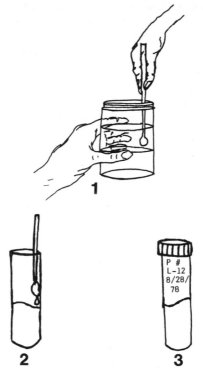

Fig. 8-10. Bacteriological sampling—swab.

6. Mark tube with identification data.
7. Send culture to lab or incubate for 24-48 hours at 37°C.

Special Considerations

• Handle swabs with care to avoid contamination.
• Mark each sample for positive identification.
• If more than 20 colonies are recovered, the level of contamination is unacceptable.

Hazards

• Spread of pathogenic organisms.

Maintenance

• Use only currently dated supplies.

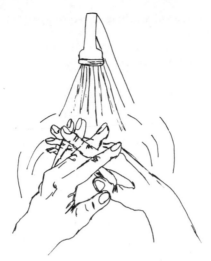

Fig. 8-11. Handwashing.

HANDWASHING TECHNIQUE

Description

Between each patient contact, RT personnel should use a handwashing technique that will minimize the harboring and transmission of microorganisms.

Objective

To remove contaminants from hands of personnel and thus prevent the possibility of cross-contamination.

Procedure

1. Approach the sink, keeping body away from it.
2. Turn on and adjust the water to a warm temperature.
3. Wet hands.
4. Apply cleaning agent.
5. Using vigorous movements, wash the hands for at least 30 seconds.
6. Rinse.
7. Repeat.

8. After the second washing, rinse well from the forearms down to the fingers.

9. Dry with paper towel.

10. Turn off water with second paper towel.

Special Considerations

- Remember to wash palms, between fingers, backs of hands, wrists and forearms.
- Use a scrubbing, circular motion when washing.
- Any personnel with an open hand cut or wound should follow this technique and use gloves for each patient.

Hazards

- Spread of microorganisms if procedure is not followed carefully.

Maintenance

- Use this procedure before and after each contact and for personal hygiene.

ASEPTIC TECHNIQUES

Description

Aseptic techniques are procedures or precautions that keep a person free from or prevent the entrance of pathogenic organisms.

Objective

To prevent the transmission of pathogens and protect the patient, the technician, and others from infection.

Procedure

Opening Packages

1. Wash hands.

2. Open package away from you.

3. Whether package is single- or double-wrapped, touch only the outside.

4. Place package on flat surface.

5. The inside of the package is sterile.

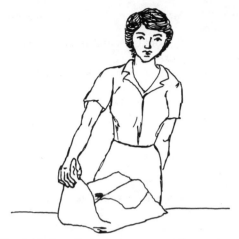

Fig. 8-12. Aseptic technique—opening packages.

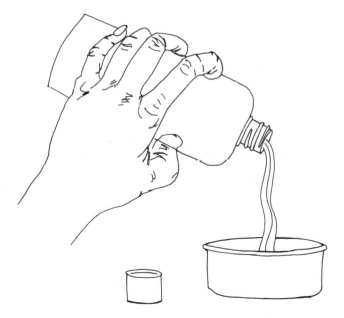

Fig. 8-13. Aseptic technique—pouring solutions.

Pouring Solutions

1. Wash hands.

2. Pick up solution container and remove cap, placing it so that inside of cap is up.

3. Pour solution into sterile container. Do not touch container with bottle.

4. Throw remainder of solution away if single use. If multiple-use container, replace cap and mark the container with date and time.

Special Considerations

- If in doubt about the sterility of an item, consider it unsterile.
- Keep sterile items separate from unsterile.
- Do not reach across a sterile field.
- The edges of all items are considered unsterile.
- Dispose of the contents of solution bottles every 24 hours or more often.

Hazards

- Contamination of supplies during preparation or use.

Maintenance

- Check dates of all supplies.
- Reprocess those supplies that become outdated.

ISOLATION TECHNIQUES

Description

Isolation techniques separate (set apart) the patient who has an infection from other patients and staff or protect the patient who is highly susceptible to infection.

Objective

To prevent the spread of infection; to prevent cross-contamination.

Procedure

See Table 8-2.

Table 8-2. Precautions

Type of Isolation	Mask	Before and After Contact Handwashing	Closed Door	Double Bagged Tissues	Double Bagged RT Equipment	Gowns	Gloves
Wound & Skin		X		X			X
Enteric		X		X			X
Respiratory	X	X	X	X	X		
Strict	X	X	X	X	X	X	X
Protective	X	X	X			X	X

Special Considerations

- When an infection is suspected, isolation techniques should be instituted. Cultures should confirm the infection.
- The type of isolation should be posted on the entrance *to the room*.
- These are not the only precautions necessary for isolation, but they represent the ones that RT personnel will most likely follow.

Hazards

- If all precautions are not followed, the infection may be transmitted.

Maintenance

- Keep the patient in isolation until cultures are negative, drainage has stopped or the patient's ability to fight infection has improved (protective isolation).

RESPIRATORY FILTERS

Description

Respiratory filters are devices that remove microorganisms from the air. Filters are used both internally and externally on respiratory therapy equipment.

CHESTER COLLEGE LIBRARY

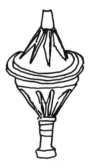

Fig. 8-14. Filters.

Objective

To remove microorganisms from the air used to power RT equipment and from the air directed to the patient from respiratory therapy equipment. To prevent cross-contamination from RT equipment.

Procedure

1. Check flow direction of filter.
2. Place external filters before the humidifier in line on main flow tubing.
3. Place external filter on supply line before the nebulizer.
4. Check resistance to air flow.
   a. Turn flow of respirator to 20 LPM.
   b. Disconnect tubing from both ends of filter.
   c. Cycle respirator to inspiration.
   d. Observe system pressure.
   e. Connect filter to machine outlet. Do not connect respirator tubing.
   f. Cycle respirator to inspiration.
   g. Observe system pressure.
   h. Difference should be less than 4 cm.H_2O.

Special Considerations

- Do not allow filters to become wet or clogged.
- Replace when recommended (see maintenance).

Hazards

- Diminish air flow with obstructed filter.
- Loss of effectiveness when filter is used longer than recommended.

Maintenance

- Use single-use filters only for one patient.
- Replace permanent filters every 500 hours, or when resistance in filter has increased (4 cm.H_2O).
- Replace internal filters at least every six months.
- Permanent filters should be steam autoclaved.

BIBLIOGRAPHY

Dixon, R. E. (ed.): Isolation Techniques for Use in Hospitals. (2nd ed.). Washington, D.C., Public Health Service, U.S. Dept. of HEW, 1975.

Lennette, E. H., Spaulding, E. H., and Truant, J. P.: Manual of Clinical Microbiology. Washington, D.C., American Society for Microbiology, 1974.

Wood, L. A., and Rambo, B.: Nursing Skills for Allied Health Personnel, Vols. 1, 2, and 3. Philadelphia, W. B. Saunders Co., 1977.

ATI BOOKLETS

Principals and Practice of Autoclave Sterilization, Principals and Practice of Ethylene Oxide Sterilization. Aseptic Thermo Indicator Company, North Hollywood, California.

PRODUCT INFORMATION

Arbrook, Inc., Arlington, Texas
Ayerst Laboratories, New York, N.Y.
Olympic Medical, Seattle, Washington

Appendix A

NAME OF TEST	NORMAL VALUES

Serum Enzyme

Alk. phosph
1.5–4.5 u./dl. adults (Bodansky) (u.=units)
5–14 u./dl. children

Acid phosph
0–1.1 u./ml. (Bodansky)

Lipase
14–280 mI.u./ml.
≤2 u./ml.

Amylase
4–25 u./ml.

SGOT
5–40 u./ml.

SGPT
5–35 u./ml.

LDH
60–100 u./ml.

CPK
55–170 u./l. males
30–135 u./l. females

Blood Values

Hematocrit
45%±7% males
40%+6% females

Hemoglobin
14–18 g.% males
12–16 g.% females
12–14 g.% children
14.5–24.5 g.% newborns

Platelet count
150,000–400,000/μl.

Erythrocytes
5×10^6/mm.^{3} (males)
4.5×10^6/mm.^{3} (females)

Leukocytes
5,000–10,000/mm.^{3}

Blood volume
69 ml./kg. males
65 ml./kg. females

Bleeding time
1–6 minutes

Prothrombin time
12–14 seconds

Blood alcohol
  Intoxication
0.3–0.4%
  Stupor
0.4–0.5%
  Coma
Above 0.5%

NAME OF TEST   NORMAL VALUES

Blood Values *(Continued)*

Serum barbituates
   Coma Phenobarbital   11 mg./100 ml.
   Others   1.5 mg./100 ml.
Serum electrolytes
   Potassium   3.5–5 mEq./l.
   Sodium   136–145 mEq./l.
   Chlorides   100–106 mEq./l.
   Bicarbonate   21–28 mEq./l.
   Phosphate   2 mEq./l.
   Sulfate   1 mEq./l.
   Organic acids   6 mEq./l.
   Calcium   5 mEq./l.
   Magnesium   2 mEq./l.

CSF

Albumin   10–30 mg./dl.
Cell count   0.8 cells/μl.
Glucose   45–75 mg./dl.
Protein total   15–45 mg./dl. (CSF)
Ventricular fluid   8–15 mg./dl.

Miscellaneous

Sweat Test
   Sodium   10–80 mEq./l.
   Chloride   4–60 mEq./l.
Urine
   *p*H   4.6–8.0
   Glucose   negative
   Acetone   negative
Blood
   Lactic acid   6–16 mg./100 ml.
   Carbon monoxide   20% Sat. produce symptoms
   *p*H   7.35–7.45
   P_{CO_2} 35–45 mm.Hg
   CO_2.   content 26–28 m.Eq./l.
   CO_2 combining power 24–29 mEq./l.
   Pa_{O_2} 95–100 mm.Hg
   O_2 capacity   16–24 vol.% (varies with Hg)
   O_2 content
      arterial   15–23 vol.%
      venous   10–16 vol.%
   O_2 saturation
      arterial   94–100%
      venous   60–85%

TEMPERATURE CONVERSION

Centigrade = Fahrenheit (0.555) − 32
Fahrenheit = Centigrade (1.8) + 32

MEASUREMENT CONVERSION

Centimeter = inches × 2.54

Inches = $\dfrac{\text{centimeter}}{2.54}$

Kilogram = pound × 2.2

Pound = $\dfrac{\text{kilogram}}{2.2}$

1 meter = 39.37 inches

GAS LAWS

P pressure
V volume
K constant
T temperature

$\dfrac{PV}{T}$ = K (Ideal Gas Law)

$\dfrac{P}{T}$ = K (Gay-Lussac's Law)

$\dfrac{V}{T}$ = K (Charles Law)

PV = K (Boyle's Law)

PULSE—NORMAL VALUES

Infants	112–130 beats/min.
Adult	70–80 beats/min.
Elderly	56–62 beats/min.

RESPIRATORY RATE—NORMAL VALUES

Infants	30–50 breaths/min.
Adults	12–20 breaths/min.

BLOOD PRESSURE—NORMAL VALUES

Infants	80/58–50/40
Adults	110/60–148/90

Table A-1. Pressure Unit Conversions

To Convert From	To	Multiply by
cm.H$_2$O	mm.Hg	0.735
	inches Hg	0.0290
	psi	0.0142
mm.Hg	cm.H$_2$O	1.36
	inches Hg	0.0394
	psi	0.0193
inches Hg	mm.Hg	25.4
	cm.H$_2$O	34.5
	psi	0.491
psi	mm.Hg	51.7
	cm.H$_2$O	70.4
	inches Hg	2.04

Appendix B

COMMONLY USED ABBREVIATIONS

GENERAL ABBREVIATIONS

Abbreviation	Meaning
a	Artery
a.c.	Before meals
ad. lib.	As needed
amt.	Amount
ant.	Anterior
approx.	Approximately (about)
b.i.d.	Twice a day
B.P.	Blood pressure
C.	Centigrade
c̄	With
cc (c.c.)	Cubic centimeters
DC	Discontinue
ECG (EKG)	Electrocardiogram (tracing of heart function)
EEG	Electroencephalogram (brain wave tracing)
E.R.	Emergency room
F.	Fahrenheit
f	Frequency
fld.	Fluid
G.I.	Gastrointestinal (stomach & intestine)
gm.	Gram (measurement)
gr.	Grain (measurement)
gtt.	Drop (measurement)
h	Hour
Hgb	Hemoglobin
H_2O	Water
h.s.	Bedtime
I and O	Intake and output
IV	Intravenous (within vein)
kg.	Kilogram (weight)
lab	Laboratory

Abbreviation	Meaning
lat.	Lateral
lb.	Pound
med.	Medial
min.	Minute
mg.	Milligram (measurement)
no.	Number
noc.	Night
NPO	Nothing by mouth (nothing per os)
O_2	Oxygen
O.B.	Obstetrics
O.R.	Operating room
p.	Pulse
Ped. or Peds, or Pedi	Pediatrics
p.o.	Per os or by mouth
postop	Postoperative (after surgery)
p.r.n.	When necessary
preop	Preoperative (before surgery)
pt.	Patient
P.T.	Physical therapist
q.d.	Every day
q.h.	Every hour
q.i.d.	Four times per day
q.o.d.	Every other day
q.s.	Quantity sufficient
r. or resp.	Respirations
Sol.	Solution
stat.	At once
sup.	Superior
tab	Tablet
TPR	Temperature, pulse, respiration
via	By way of
wt.	Weight

RESPIRATORY ABBREVIATIONS

Abbreviation		Example
A	alveolar gas	$P_{A_{O_2}}$
B	barometric	P_B
D	dead space gas	V_D
E	Expired gas	$P_{E_{CO_2}}$
I	Inspired gas	$F_{I_{O_2}}$
a	arterial blood	Pa_{O_2}
b	blood	$\dot{Q}b$
c	capillary blood	$P_{C_{O_2}}$
v	venous blood	Pv_{CO_2}
$\bar{v}$	mixed venous blood	$P\bar{v}_{CO_2}$

	Abbreviation	Example
C	concentration of gas	Ca_{O_2}
F	fractional concentration of gas	$F_{E_{CO_2}}$
P	pressure of gas	Pa_{O_2}
Q	blood volume	
V	gas volume	
$\dot{Q}$	blood flow rate	$\dot{Q}b$
$\dot{V}$	gas flow rate	$\dot{V}_A$
S	saturation	Sa_{O_2}
T.V.		tidal volume
f		frequency
M.V.		minute ventilation

Appendix C

Apnea. Cessation of ventilation in the resting expiratory position.

Apneusis. Cessation of ventilation in the inspiratory position.

Apneustic breathing. Apneusis interrupted periodically by expiration. May be rhythmic, e.g., brain stem.

Breathing. Alternating inspiration and expiration of air into and out of the lungs.

Breathing cycle. From end expiration to end expiration.

Breathing frequency. Number of breathing cycles per unit of time.

Breathing pattern. Refers to the characteristics of the ventilatory activity.

Biots breathing. Alternate hypernea (either T.V. or f) and apnea occur in abrupt attacks for regular periods, e.g. lesions of medulla meningitis.

Cheyne–Stokes breathing. Pattern of breathing in which tidal volume first progressively increases and then progressively decreases, followed by a period of apnea, then breathing sequence is repeated, e.g., cardiac decompensation or cerebral terminal anoxia.

Dyspnea. Difficult or labored breathing—subjective feeling of shortness of breath.

Eupnea. Normal spontaneous breathing.

Gasp. A ventilatory movement consisting of a sudden brief inspiratory effort.

Hypernea. Increased breathing—usually refers to increased tidal volume with or without increased frequency.

Hyperventilation. Pulmonary ventilation exceeds the metabolic rate for respiratory gas exchange. (T.V. or f or both).

Hyponea. Decreased breathing (T.V. or f).

Hypoventilation. Pulmonary ventilation less than the metabolic rate for respiratory gas exchange (T.V. or f or both).

Kussmaul breathing. Inspirations are forced and regular but expiration unaffected, e.g., diabetic acidosis.

Orthopnea. Dyspnea that can be relieved by sitting in upright position.

Pant. Rapid shallow breathing.

Respiration. Gas exchange:

external—between lungs and pulmonary circulatory system.

internal—between arterial system and cell.

Tachypnea. Increased frequency of breathing (polypnea).

Ventilation. Volume of air moved into and out of the lungs per unit of time.

$$f \times V_T = M.V.$$

$$\text{many}^{\text{how}} \times \text{much}^{\text{how}} = \text{total}$$

BIBLIOGRAPHY

Brooks, S. M.: Integrated Basic Science. St. Louis, C. V. Mosby Co., 1976.

Davidsohn, I., and Henry, J. B.: Clinical Diagnosis by Laboratory Methods. Philadelphia, W. B. Saunders, 1974.

Slonim, N. B. and Hamilton, L. H.: Respiratory Physiology. St. Louis, C. V. Mosby Co., 1976.

(Adapted from: Slonim, N. B., and Hamilton, L. H.: Respiratory Physiology. St. Louis, C. V. Mosby, 1976.)

Index

Index

Numerals in *italics* indicate a figure; "t" following a page number indicates a table.